Healin' Vibes

A cannabis logbook

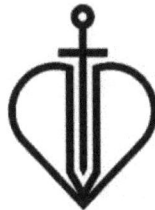

WELLNESS WARRIOR PRESS
www.wellnesswarriorpress.com

ISBN: 978-1-990271-10-6
Copyright © 2021 by Wellness Warrior Press

This journal belongs to...

_____

My Health

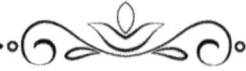

diagnosis	date

SYMPTOMS I HOPE TO RELIEVE WITH CANNABIS

TREATMENT PLAN / DAILY DOSING

CURRENT MEDICATION(S)

name	*dose*	hoping to stop / reduce	
		☐ Yes	☐ No
		☐ Yes	☐ No
		☐ Yes	☐ No
		☐ Yes	☐ No
		☐ Yes	☐ No
		☐ Yes	☐ No
		☐ Yes	☐ No
		☐ Yes	☐ No
		☐ Yes	☐ No
		☐ Yes	☐ No
		☐ Yes	☐ No
		☐ Yes	☐ No
		☐ Yes	☐ No
		☐ Yes	☐ No
		☐ Yes	☐ No
		☐ Yes	☐ No
		☐ Yes	☐ No
		☐ Yes	☐ No

Note: never attempt to stop or reduce your medication(s) without first consulting with your physician.

DOCTOR / SPECIALIST INFORMATION

Name	Address	Contact

Summary

For each cannabis use, return to this summary page and document your rating (1 – 5)

#	Rating	#	Rating	#	Rating	#	Rating
1		31		61		91	
2		32		62		92	
3		33		63		93	
4		34		64		94	
5		35		65		95	
6		36		66		96	
7		37		67		97	
8		38		68		98	
9		39		69		99	
10		40		70		100	
11		41		71		101	
12		42		72		102	
13		43		73		103	
14		44		74		104	
15		45		75		105	
16		46		76		106	
17		47		77		107	
18		48		78		108	
19		49		79		109	
20		50		80		110	
21		51		81		111	
22		52		82		112	
23		53		83		113	
24		54		84		114	
25		55		85		115	
26		56		86		116	
27		57		87		117	
28		58		88		118	
29		59		89		119	
30		60		90		120	

Distributors

#1

Name: _____ ☐ **Favorite**

Address:_____

Contact:_____

☐ Friendly   ☐ Clean   ☐ Knowledgeable

☐ Professional   ☐ Fair prices   ☐ Quality Products

Notes: _____

MY RATING: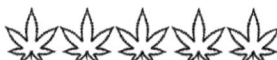

#2

Name: _____ ☐ **Favorite**

Address:_____

Contact:_____

☐ Friendly   ☐ Clean   ☐ Knowledgeable

☐ Professional   ☐ Fair prices   ☐ Quality Products

Notes: _____

MY RATING: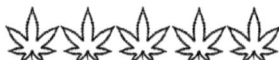

#3

Name: _____ ☐ **Favorite**

Address:_____

Contact:_____

☐ Friendly   ☐ Clean   ☐ Knowledgeable

☐ Professional   ☐ Fair prices   ☐ Quality Products

Notes: _____

MY RATING: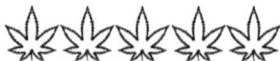

#4

Name: _____ ☐ **Favorite**

Address:_____

Contact:_____

☐ Friendly   ☐ Clean   ☐ Knowledgeable

☐ Professional   ☐ Fair prices   ☐ Quality Products

Notes: _____

MY RATING: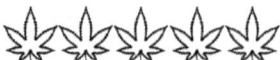

Distributors — cont'd

#5

Name: _____ ☐ **Favorite**

Address:_____

Contact:_____

☐ Friendly   ☐ Clean   ☐ Knowledgeable

☐ Professional ☐ Fair prices ☐ Quality Products

Notes: _____

MY RATING: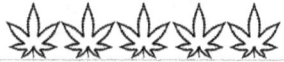

#6

Name: _____ ☐ **Favorite**

Address:_____

Contact:_____

☐ Friendly   ☐ Clean   ☐ Knowledgeable

☐ Professional ☐ Fair prices ☐ Quality Products

Notes: _____

MY RATING: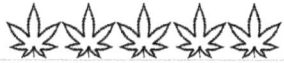

#7

Name: _____ ☐ **Favorite**

Address:_____

Contact:_____

☐ Friendly   ☐ Clean   ☐ Knowledgeable

☐ Professional ☐ Fair prices ☐ Quality Products

Notes: _____

MY RATING: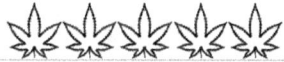

#8

Name: _____ ☐ **Favorite**

Address:_____

Contact:_____

☐ Friendly   ☐ Clean   ☐ Knowledgeable

☐ Professional ☐ Fair prices ☐ Quality Products

Notes: _____

MY RATING: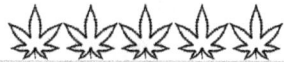

DATE:		ENTRY:	1

Strain:_____ Distributor:_____

PRICE: _____
TOTAL ACQUIRED: _____
PURCHASE DATE: _____
DISTRIBUTOR #: _____

description / notes

DOSAGE / INSTRUCTIONS	CERTIFICATE OF ANALYSIS	
	☐ Yes	☐ No

FORM
☐ Flower
☐ Edible
☐ Oil
☐ Tincture
☐ _____

METHOD
☐ Smoked
☐ Vaped
☐ Ingested
☐ Topical
☐ _____

CONTENT
_____% CBD
_____% THC
_____% _____
_____% _____
_____% _____

VARIETY
☐ Indica
☐ Sativa
☐ Hybrid

Dose: _____   Smell / Taste: _____

Time to take effect: _____   Effect duration: _____

Reliefs

Pain: ① ② ③ ④ ⑤   Stress: ① ② ③ ④ ⑤
Nausea: ① ② ③ ④ ⑤   Anxiety: ① ② ③ ④ ⑤
Inflammation: ① ② ③ ④ ⑤   Depression: ① ② ③ ④ ⑤
Appetite: ① ② ③ ④ ⑤   Insomnia: ① ② ③ ④ ⑤

Other positive effects: _____

Adverse effects

Anxiety: ① ② ③ ④ ⑤   Dry Mouth: ① ② ③ ④ ⑤
Munchies: ① ② ③ ④ ⑤   Fatigue: ① ② ③ ④ ⑤

Other adverse effects: _____

Notes

My Rating: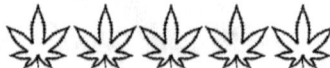

Strain:_____ Distributor:_____

PRICE: _____

TOTAL ACQUIRED: _____

PURCHASE DATE: _____

DISTRIBUTOR #: _____

description / notes

DOSAGE / INSTRUCTIONS	CERTIFICATE OF ANALYSIS	
	☐ Yes	☐ No

FORM
☐ Flower
☐ Edible
☐ Oil
☐ Tincture
☐ _____

METHOD
☐ Smoked
☐ Vaped
☐ Ingested
☐ Topical
☐ _____

CONTENT
_____% CBD
_____% THC
_____% _____
_____% _____
_____% _____

VARIETY
☐ Indica
☐ Sativa
☐ Hybrid

Dose: _____ Smell / Taste: _____

Time to take effect: _____ Effect duration: _____

Reliefs

Pain: ① ② ③ ④ ⑤   Stress: ① ② ③ ④ ⑤

Nausea: ① ② ③ ④ ⑤   Anxiety: ① ② ③ ④ ⑤

Inflammation: ① ② ③ ④ ⑤   Insomnia: ① ② ③ ④ ⑤

Appetite: ① ② ③ ④ ⑤   Depression: ① ② ③ ④ ⑤

Other positive effects: _____

Adverse effects

Anxiety: ① ② ③ ④ ⑤   Dry Mouth: ① ② ③ ④ ⑤

Munchies: ① ② ③ ④ ⑤   Fatigue: ① ② ③ ④ ⑤

Other adverse effects: _____

Notes

_____

_____

My Rating: 🍁 🍁 🍁 🍁 🍁

DATE:	ENTRY:	3

Strain:_____ Distributor:_____

PRICE: _____

TOTAL ACQUIRED: _____

PURCHASE DATE: _____

DISTRIBUTOR #: _____

description / notes

DOSAGE / INSTRUCTIONS	CERTIFICATE OF ANALYSIS	
	☐ Yes	☐ No

FORM
☐ Flower
☐ Edible
☐ Oil
☐ Tincture
☐ _____

METHOD
☐ Smoked
☐ Vaped
☐ Ingested
☐ Topical
☐ _____

CONTENT
_____% CBD
_____% THC
_____% _____
_____% _____
_____% _____

VARIETY
☐ Indica
☐ Sativa
☐ Hybrid

Dose: _____ Smell / Taste: _____

Time to take effect: _____ Effect duration: _____

Reliefs

Pain:	①	②	③	④	⑤	Stress:	①	②	③	④	⑤
Nausea:	①	②	③	④	⑤	Anxiety:	①	②	③	④	⑤
Inflammation:	①	②	③	④	⑤	Insomnia:	①	②	③	④	⑤
Appetite:	①	②	③	④	⑤	Depression:	①	②	③	④	⑤

Other positive effects: _____

Adverse effects

Anxiety:	①	②	③	④	⑤	Dry Mouth:	①	②	③	④	⑤
Munchies:	①	②	③	④	⑤	Fatigue:	①	②	③	④	⑤

Other adverse effects: _____

Notes

My Rating: 🍁🍁🍁🍁🍁

Strain:_____ Distributor:_____

PRICE: _____

TOTAL ACQUIRED: _____

PURCHASE DATE: _____

DISTRIBUTOR #: _____

description / notes

DOSAGE / INSTRUCTIONS	CERTIFICATE OF ANALYSIS	
	☐ Yes	☐ No

FORM
☐ Flower
☐ Edible
☐ Oil
☐ Tincture
☐ _____

METHOD
☐ Smoked
☐ Vaped
☐ Ingested
☐ Topical
☐ _____

CONTENT
____% CBD
____% THC
____% ____
____% ____
____% ____

VARIETY
☐ Indica
☐ Sativa
☐ Hybrid

Dose: _____ Smell / Taste: _____

Time to take effect: _____ Effect duration: _____

Reliefs

Pain: ① ② ③ ④ ⑤   Stress: ① ② ③ ④ ⑤

Nausea: ① ② ③ ④ ⑤   Anxiety: ① ② ③ ④ ⑤

Inflammation: ① ② ③ ④ ⑤   Insomnia: ① ② ③ ④ ⑤

Appetite: ① ② ③ ④ ⑤   Depression: ① ② ③ ④ ⑤

Other positive effects: _____

Adverse effects

Anxiety: ① ② ③ ④ ⑤   Dry Mouth: ① ② ③ ④ ⑤

Munchies: ① ② ③ ④ ⑤   Fatigue: ① ② ③ ④ ⑤

Other adverse effects: _____

Notes
_____

My Rating: 🍁 🍁 🍁 🍁 🍁

Strain:_____ Distributor:_____

PRICE:	_____	
TOTAL ACQUIRED:	_____	*description / notes*
PURCHASE DATE:	_____	
DISTRIBUTOR #:	_____	

DOSAGE / INSTRUCTIONS	CERTIFICATE OF ANALYSIS	
	☐ Yes	☐ No

FORM	METHOD	CONTENT	VARIETY
☐ Flower	☐ Smoked	_____% CBD	☐ Indica
☐ Edible	☐ Vaped	_____% THC	☐ Sativa
☐ Oil	☐ Ingested	_____% _____	☐ Hybrid
☐ Tincture	☐ Topical	_____% _____	
☐ _____	☐ _____	_____% _____	

Dose: _____ Smell / Taste: _____

Time to take effect: _____ Effect duration: _____

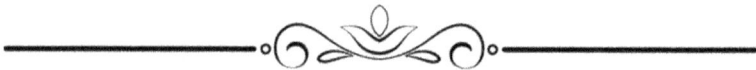

Reliefs

Pain:	① ② ③ ④ ⑤	Stress:	① ② ③ ④ ⑤
Nausea:	① ② ③ ④ ⑤	Anxiety:	① ② ③ ④ ⑤
Inflammation:	① ② ③ ④ ⑤	Insomnia:	① ② ③ ④ ⑤
Appetite:	① ② ③ ④ ⑤	Depression:	① ② ③ ④ ⑤

Other positive effects: _____

Adverse effects

Anxiety:	① ② ③ ④ ⑤	Dry Mouth:	① ② ③ ④ ⑤
Munchies:	① ② ③ ④ ⑤	Fatigue:	① ② ③ ④ ⑤

Other adverse effects: _____

Notes

My Rating: 🌿 🌿 🌿 🌿 🌿

DATE:		ENTRY:	6

Strain:_____ Distributor:_____

PRICE: _____
TOTAL ACQUIRED: _____
PURCHASE DATE: _____
DISTRIBUTOR #: _____

description / notes

DOSAGE / INSTRUCTIONS	CERTIFICATE OF ANALYSIS	
	☐ Yes	☐ No

FORM
☐ Flower
☐ Edible
☐ Oil
☐ Tincture
☐ _____

METHOD
☐ Smoked
☐ Vaped
☐ Ingested
☐ Topical
☐ _____

CONTENT
_____% CBD
_____% THC
_____% _____
_____% _____
_____% _____

VARIETY
☐ Indica
☐ Sativa
☐ Hybrid

Dose: _____ Smell / Taste: _____

Time to take effect: _____ Effect duration: _____

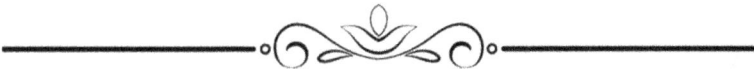

Reliefs

Pain:	① ② ③ ④ ⑤		Stress:	① ② ③ ④ ⑤
Nausea:	① ② ③ ④ ⑤		Anxiety:	① ② ③ ④ ⑤
Inflammation:	① ② ③ ④ ⑤		Insomnia:	① ② ③ ④ ⑤
Appetite:	① ② ③ ④ ⑤		Depression:	① ② ③ ④ ⑤

Other positive effects: _____

Adverse effects

Anxiety:	① ② ③ ④ ⑤		Dry Mouth:	① ② ③ ④ ⑤
Munchies:	① ② ③ ④ ⑤		Fatigue:	① ② ③ ④ ⑤

Other adverse effects: _____

Notes

My Rating: 🍁 🍁 🍁 🍁 🍁

DATE:		ENTRY:	7

Strain:_____ Distributor:_____

PRICE: _____

TOTAL ACQUIRED: _____

PURCHASE DATE: _____

DISTRIBUTOR #: _____

description / notes

DOSAGE / INSTRUCTIONS	CERTIFICATE OF ANALYSIS	
	☐ Yes	☐ No

FORM
☐ Flower
☐ Edible
☐ Oil
☐ Tincture
☐ _____

METHOD
☐ Smoked
☐ Vaped
☐ Ingested
☐ Topical
☐ _____

CONTENT
_____% CBD
_____% THC
_____% _____
_____% _____
_____% _____

VARIETY
☐ Indica
☐ Sativa
☐ Hybrid

Dose: _____ Smell / Taste: _____

Time to take effect: _____ Effect duration: _____

Reliefs

Pain:	① ② ③ ④ ⑤	Stress:	① ② ③ ④ ⑤
Nausea:	① ② ③ ④ ⑤	Anxiety:	① ② ③ ④ ⑤
Inflammation:	① ② ③ ④ ⑤	Insomnia:	① ② ③ ④ ⑤
Appetite:	① ② ③ ④ ⑤	Depression:	① ② ③ ④ ⑤

Other positive effects: _____

Adverse effects

Anxiety:	① ② ③ ④ ⑤	Dry Mouth:	① ② ③ ④ ⑤
Munchies:	① ② ③ ④ ⑤	Fatigue:	① ② ③ ④ ⑤

Other adverse effects: _____

Notes

My Rating:

Strain:_____ Distributor:_____

PRICE: _____

TOTAL ACQUIRED: _____

PURCHASE DATE: _____

DISTRIBUTOR #: _____

description / notes

DOSAGE / INSTRUCTIONS	CERTIFICATE OF ANALYSIS	
	☐ Yes	☐ No

FORM
- ☐ Flower
- ☐ Edible
- ☐ Oil
- ☐ Tincture
- ☐ _____

METHOD
- ☐ Smoked
- ☐ Vaped
- ☐ Ingested
- ☐ Topical
- ☐ _____

CONTENT
- ____% CBD
- ____% THC
- ____% ____
- ____% ____
- ____% ____

VARIETY
- ☐ Indica
- ☐ Sativa
- ☐ Hybrid

Dose: _____ Smell / Taste: _____

Time to take effect: _____ Effect duration: _____

Reliefs

Pain:	①	②	③	④	⑤	Stress:	①	②	③	④	⑤
Nausea:	①	②	③	④	⑤	Anxiety:	①	②	③	④	⑤
Inflammation:	①	②	③	④	⑤	Insomnia:	①	②	③	④	⑤
Appetite:	①	②	③	④	⑤	Depression:	①	②	③	④	⑤

Other positive effects: _____

Adverse effects

Anxiety:	①	②	③	④	⑤	Dry Mouth:	①	②	③	④	⑤
Munchies:	①	②	③	④	⑤	Fatigue:	①	②	③	④	⑤

Other adverse effects: _____

Notes

My Rating: ✿ ✿ ✿ ✿ ✿

DATE:	ENTRY:	9

Strain:_____ Distributor:_____

PRICE: _____

TOTAL ACQUIRED: _____

PURCHASE DATE: _____

DISTRIBUTOR #: _____

description / notes

DOSAGE / INSTRUCTIONS	CERTIFICATE OF ANALYSIS	
	☐ Yes	☐ No

FORM
☐ Flower
☐ Edible
☐ Oil
☐ Tincture
☐ _____

METHOD
☐ Smoked
☐ Vaped
☐ Ingested
☐ Topical
☐ _____

CONTENT
_____% CBD
_____% THC
_____% _____
_____% _____
_____% _____

VARIETY
☐ Indica
☐ Sativa
☐ Hybrid

Dose: _____   Smell / Taste: _____

Time to take effect: _____   Effect duration: _____

Reliefs

Pain:	① ② ③ ④ ⑤	Stress:	① ② ③ ④ ⑤
Nausea:	① ② ③ ④ ⑤	Anxiety:	① ② ③ ④ ⑤
Inflammation:	① ② ③ ④ ⑤	Insomnia:	① ② ③ ④ ⑤
Appetite:	① ② ③ ④ ⑤	Depression:	① ② ③ ④ ⑤

Other positive effects: _____

Adverse effects

Anxiety:	① ② ③ ④ ⑤	Dry Mouth:	① ② ③ ④ ⑤
Munchies:	① ② ③ ④ ⑤	Fatigue:	① ② ③ ④ ⑤

Other adverse effects: _____

Notes

My Rating: 🍁 🍁 🍁 🍁 🍁

DATE:	ENTRY:	10

Strain:_____ Distributor:_____

PRICE: _____
TOTAL ACQUIRED: _____
PURCHASE DATE: _____
DISTRIBUTOR #: _____

description / notes

DOSAGE / INSTRUCTIONS	CERTIFICATE OF ANALYSIS	
	☐ Yes	☐ No

FORM
☐ Flower
☐ Edible
☐ Oil
☐ Tincture
☐ _____

METHOD
☐ Smoked
☐ Vaped
☐ Ingested
☐ Topical
☐ _____

CONTENT
_____% CBD
_____% THC
_____% _____
_____% _____
_____% _____

VARIETY
☐ Indica
☐ Sativa
☐ Hybrid

Dose: _____ Smell / Taste: _____

Time to take effect: _____ Effect duration: _____

Reliefs
Pain: ① ② ③ ④ ⑤   Stress: ① ② ③ ④ ⑤
Nausea: ① ② ③ ④ ⑤   Anxiety: ① ② ③ ④ ⑤
Inflammation: ① ② ③ ④ ⑤   Insomnia: ① ② ③ ④ ⑤
Appetite: ① ② ③ ④ ⑤   Depression: ① ② ③ ④ ⑤

Other positive effects: _____

Adverse effects
Anxiety: ① ② ③ ④ ⑤   Dry Mouth: ① ② ③ ④ ⑤
Munchies: ① ② ③ ④ ⑤   Fatigue: ① ② ③ ④ ⑤

Other adverse effects: _____

Notes

My Rating: 🍁 🍁 🍁 🍁 🍁

DATE:	ENTRY:	11

Strain:_____ Distributor:_____

PRICE: _____
TOTAL ACQUIRED: _____
PURCHASE DATE: _____
DISTRIBUTOR #: _____

description / notes

DOSAGE / INSTRUCTIONS	CERTIFICATE OF ANALYSIS	
	☐ Yes	☐ No

FORM	METHOD	CONTENT	VARIETY
☐ Flower	☐ Smoked	____% CBD	☐ Indica
☐ Edible	☐ Vaped	____% THC	☐ Sativa
☐ Oil	☐ Ingested	____% ____	☐ Hybrid
☐ Tincture	☐ Topical	____% ____	
☐ _____	☐ _____	____% ____	

Dose: _____ Smell / Taste: _____

Time to take effect: _____ Effect duration: _____

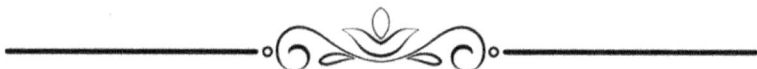

Reliefs

Pain:	① ② ③ ④ ⑤	Stress:	① ② ③ ④ ⑤
Nausea:	① ② ③ ④ ⑤	Anxiety:	① ② ③ ④ ⑤
Inflammation:	① ② ③ ④ ⑤	Insomnia:	① ② ③ ④ ⑤
Appetite:	① ② ③ ④ ⑤	Depression:	① ② ③ ④ ⑤

Other positive effects: _____

Adverse effects

Anxiety:	① ② ③ ④ ⑤	Dry Mouth:	① ② ③ ④ ⑤
Munchies:	① ② ③ ④ ⑤	Fatigue:	① ② ③ ④ ⑤

Other adverse effects: _____

Notes

My Rating: 🍁 🍁 🍁 🍁 🍁

DATE:		ENTRY:	12

Strain:_____ Distributor:_____

PRICE: _____

TOTAL ACQUIRED: _____

PURCHASE DATE: _____

DISTRIBUTOR #: _____

description / notes

DOSAGE / INSTRUCTIONS	CERTIFICATE OF ANALYSIS	
	☐ Yes	☐ No

FORM
☐ Flower
☐ Edible
☐ Oil
☐ Tincture
☐ _____

METHOD
☐ Smoked
☐ Vaped
☐ Ingested
☐ Topical
☐ _____

CONTENT
_____% CBD
_____% THC
_____% _____
_____% _____
_____% _____

VARIETY
☐ Indica
☐ Sativa
☐ Hybrid

Dose: _____ Smell / Taste: _____

Time to take effect: _____ Effect duration: _____

Reliefs

Pain:	① ② ③ ④ ⑤	Stress:	① ② ③ ④ ⑤
Nausea:	① ② ③ ④ ⑤	Anxiety:	① ② ③ ④ ⑤
Inflammation:	① ② ③ ④ ⑤	Insomnia:	① ② ③ ④ ⑤
Appetite:	① ② ③ ④ ⑤	Depression:	① ② ③ ④ ⑤

Other positive effects: _____

Adverse effects

Anxiety:	① ② ③ ④ ⑤	Dry Mouth:	① ② ③ ④ ⑤
Munchies:	① ② ③ ④ ⑤	Fatigue:	① ② ③ ④ ⑤

Other adverse effects: _____

Notes

_____

_____

My Rating: ✿ ✿ ✿ ✿ ✿

DATE:		ENTRY:	13

Strain:_____ Distributor:_____

PRICE: _____
TOTAL ACQUIRED: _____
PURCHASE DATE: _____
DISTRIBUTOR #: _____

description / notes

DOSAGE / INSTRUCTIONS	CERTIFICATE OF ANALYSIS	
	☐ Yes	☐ No

FORM
☐ Flower
☐ Edible
☐ Oil
☐ Tincture
☐ _____

METHOD
☐ Smoked
☐ Vaped
☐ Ingested
☐ Topical
☐ _____

CONTENT
_____% CBD
_____% THC
_____% _____
_____% _____
_____% _____

VARIETY
☐ Indica
☐ Sativa
☐ Hybrid

Dose: _____   Smell / Taste: _____

Time to take effect: _____   Effect duration: _____

Reliefs

Pain:	①	②	③	④	⑤	Stress:	①	②	③	④	⑤
Nausea:	①	②	③	④	⑤	Anxiety:	①	②	③	④	⑤
Inflammation:	①	②	③	④	⑤	Insomnia:	①	②	③	④	⑤
Appetite:	①	②	③	④	⑤	Depression:	①	②	③	④	⑤

Other positive effects: _____

Adverse effects

Anxiety:	①	②	③	④	⑤	Dry Mouth:	①	②	③	④	⑤
Munchies:	①	②	③	④	⑤	Fatigue:	①	②	③	④	⑤

Other adverse effects: _____

Notes

My Rating: 🍁 🍁 🍁 🍁 🍁

DATE:		ENTRY:	14

Strain:_____ Distributor:_____

PRICE: _____	*description / notes*
TOTAL ACQUIRED: _____	
PURCHASE DATE: _____	
DISTRIBUTOR #: _____	

DOSAGE / INSTRUCTIONS	CERTIFICATE OF ANALYSIS	
	☐ Yes	☐ No

FORM	METHOD	CONTENT	VARIETY
☐ Flower	☐ Smoked	____% CBD	☐ Indica
☐ Edible	☐ Vaped	____% THC	☐ Sativa
☐ Oil	☐ Ingested	____% _____	☐ Hybrid
☐ Tincture	☐ Topical	____% _____	
☐ _____	☐ _____	____% _____	

Dose: _____ Smell / Taste: _____

Time to take effect: _____ Effect duration: _____

Reliefs

Pain: ① ② ③ ④ ⑤		Stress: ① ② ③ ④ ⑤	
Nausea: ① ② ③ ④ ⑤		Anxiety: ① ② ③ ④ ⑤	
Inflammation: ① ② ③ ④ ⑤		Insomnia: ① ② ③ ④ ⑤	
Appetite: ① ② ③ ④ ⑤		Depression: ① ② ③ ④ ⑤	

Other positive effects: _____

Adverse effects

Anxiety: ① ② ③ ④ ⑤		Dry Mouth: ① ② ③ ④ ⑤	
Munchies: ① ② ③ ④ ⑤		Fatigue: ① ② ③ ④ ⑤	

Other adverse effects: _____

Notes

My Rating: 🌿 🌿 🌿 🌿 🌿

Strain:_____ Distributor:_____

PRICE: _____

TOTAL ACQUIRED: _____

PURCHASE DATE: _____

DISTRIBUTOR #: _____

description / notes

DOSAGE / INSTRUCTIONS	CERTIFICATE OF ANALYSIS	
	☐ Yes	☐ No

FORM	METHOD	CONTENT	VARIETY
☐ Flower	☐ Smoked	____% CBD	☐ Indica
☐ Edible	☐ Vaped	____% THC	☐ Sativa
☐ Oil	☐ Ingested	____% ____	☐ Hybrid
☐ Tincture	☐ Topical	____% ____	
☐ _____	☐ _____	____% ____	

Dose: _____ Smell / Taste: _____

Time to take effect: _____ Effect duration: _____

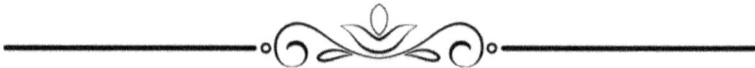

Reliefs

Pain: ①②③④⑤   Stress: ①②③④⑤

Nausea: ①②③④⑤   Anxiety: ①②③④⑤

Inflammation: ①②③④⑤   Insomnia: ①②③④⑤

Appetite: ①②③④⑤   Depression: ①②③④⑤

Other positive effects: _____

Adverse effects

Anxiety: ①②③④⑤   Dry Mouth: ①②③④⑤

Munchies: ①②③④⑤   Fatigue: ①②③④⑤

Other adverse effects: _____

Notes

My Rating: 🍁🍁🍁🍁🍁

DATE:	ENTRY:	16

Strain:_____ Distributor:_____

PRICE: _____	description / notes
TOTAL ACQUIRED: _____	
PURCHASE DATE: _____	
DISTRIBUTOR #: _____	

DOSAGE / INSTRUCTIONS	CERTIFICATE OF ANALYSIS	
	☐ Yes	☐ No

FORM	METHOD	CONTENT	VARIETY
☐ Flower	☐ Smoked	_____% CBD	☐ Indica
☐ Edible	☐ Vaped	_____% THC	☐ Sativa
☐ Oil	☐ Ingested	_____% _____	☐ Hybrid
☐ Tincture	☐ Topical	_____% _____	
☐ _____	☐ _____	_____% _____	

Dose: _____ Smell / Taste: _____

Time to take effect: _____ Effect duration: _____

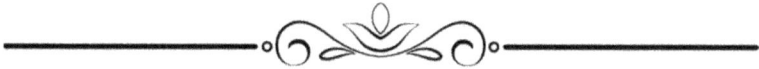

Reliefs

Pain:	① ② ③ ④ ⑤	Stress:	① ② ③ ④ ⑤
Nausea:	① ② ③ ④ ⑤	Anxiety:	① ② ③ ④ ⑤
Inflammation:	① ② ③ ④ ⑤	Insomnia:	① ② ③ ④ ⑤
Appetite:	① ② ③ ④ ⑤	Depression:	① ② ③ ④ ⑤

Other positive effects: _____

Adverse effects

Anxiety:	① ② ③ ④ ⑤	Dry Mouth:	① ② ③ ④ ⑤
Munchies:	① ② ③ ④ ⑤	Fatigue:	① ② ③ ④ ⑤

Other adverse effects: _____

Notes

My Rating: 🍁 🍁 🍁 🍁 🍁

DATE:	ENTRY:	17

Strain:_____ Distributor:_____

PRICE: _____
TOTAL ACQUIRED: _____
PURCHASE DATE: _____
DISTRIBUTOR #: _____

description / notes

DOSAGE / INSTRUCTIONS	CERTIFICATE OF ANALYSIS	
	☐ Yes	☐ No

FORM
☐ Flower
☐ Edible
☐ Oil
☐ Tincture
☐ _____

METHOD
☐ Smoked
☐ Vaped
☐ Ingested
☐ Topical
☐ _____

CONTENT
_____% CBD
_____% THC
_____% _____
_____% _____
_____% _____

VARIETY
☐ Indica
☐ Sativa
☐ Hybrid

Dose: _____ Smell / Taste: _____

Time to take effect: _____ Effect duration: _____

Reliefs

Pain: ① ② ③ ④ ⑤   Stress: ① ② ③ ④ ⑤
Nausea: ① ② ③ ④ ⑤   Anxiety: ① ② ③ ④ ⑤
Inflammation: ① ② ③ ④ ⑤   Insomnia: ① ② ③ ④ ⑤
Appetite: ① ② ③ ④ ⑤   Depression: ① ② ③ ④ ⑤

Other positive effects: _____

Adverse effects

Anxiety: ① ② ③ ④ ⑤   Dry Mouth: ① ② ③ ④ ⑤
Munchies: ① ② ③ ④ ⑤   Fatigue: ① ② ③ ④ ⑤

Other adverse effects: _____

Notes

My Rating: 🍁 🍁 🍁 🍁 🍁

DATE:	ENTRY:	18

Strain:_____ Distributor:_____

PRICE: _____

TOTAL ACQUIRED: _____

PURCHASE DATE: _____

DISTRIBUTOR #: _____

description / notes

DOSAGE / INSTRUCTIONS	CERTIFICATE OF ANALYSIS	
	☐ Yes	☐ No

FORM
☐ Flower
☐ Edible
☐ Oil
☐ Tincture
☐ _____

METHOD
☐ Smoked
☐ Vaped
☐ Ingested
☐ Topical
☐ _____

CONTENT
_____% CBD
_____% THC
_____% _____
_____% _____
_____% _____

VARIETY
☐ Indica
☐ Sativa
☐ Hybrid

Dose: _____ Smell / Taste: _____

Time to take effect: _____ Effect duration: _____

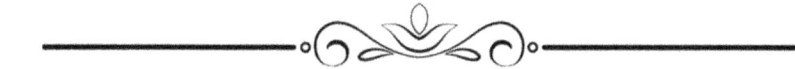

Reliefs

Pain: ① ② ③ ④ ⑤	Stress: ① ② ③ ④ ⑤
Nausea: ① ② ③ ④ ⑤	Anxiety: ① ② ③ ④ ⑤
Inflammation: ① ② ③ ④ ⑤	Insomnia: ① ② ③ ④ ⑤
Appetite: ① ② ③ ④ ⑤	Depression: ① ② ③ ④ ⑤

Other positive effects: _____

Adverse effects

Anxiety: ① ② ③ ④ ⑤	Dry Mouth: ① ② ③ ④ ⑤
Munchies: ① ② ③ ④ ⑤	Fatigue: ① ② ③ ④ ⑤

Other adverse effects: _____

Notes

My Rating: ✴ ✴ ✴ ✴ ✴

Strain:_____ Distributor:_____

PRICE: _____
TOTAL ACQUIRED: _____
PURCHASE DATE: _____
DISTRIBUTOR #: _____

description / notes

DOSAGE / INSTRUCTIONS	CERTIFICATE OF ANALYSIS	
	☐ Yes	☐ No

FORM
☐ Flower
☐ Edible
☐ Oil
☐ Tincture
☐ _____

METHOD
☐ Smoked
☐ Vaped
☐ Ingested
☐ Topical
☐ _____

CONTENT
_____% CBD
_____% THC
_____% _____
_____% _____
_____% _____

VARIETY
☐ Indica
☐ Sativa
☐ Hybrid

Dose: _____ Smell / Taste: _____

Time to take effect: _____ Effect duration: _____

Reliefs

Pain: ① ② ③ ④ ⑤   Stress: ① ② ③ ④ ⑤
Nausea: ① ② ③ ④ ⑤   Anxiety: ① ② ③ ④ ⑤
Inflammation: ① ② ③ ④ ⑤   Insomnia: ① ② ③ ④ ⑤
Appetite: ① ② ③ ④ ⑤   Depression: ① ② ③ ④ ⑤

Other positive effects: _____

Adverse effects

Anxiety: ① ② ③ ④ ⑤   Dry Mouth: ① ② ③ ④ ⑤
Munchies: ① ② ③ ④ ⑤   Fatigue: ① ② ③ ④ ⑤

Other adverse effects: _____

Notes

My Rating: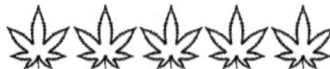

DATE:	ENTRY:	20

Strain:_____ Distributor:_____

PRICE: _____

TOTAL ACQUIRED: _____

PURCHASE DATE: _____

DISTRIBUTOR #: _____

description / notes

DOSAGE / INSTRUCTIONS	CERTIFICATE OF ANALYSIS	
	☐ Yes	☐ No

FORM
☐ Flower
☐ Edible
☐ Oil
☐ Tincture
☐ _____

METHOD
☐ Smoked
☐ Vaped
☐ Ingested
☐ Topical
☐ _____

CONTENT
_____% CBD
_____% THC
_____% _____
_____% _____
_____% _____

VARIETY
☐ Indica
☐ Sativa
☐ Hybrid

Dose: _____   Smell / Taste: _____

Time to take effect: _____   Effect duration: _____

Reliefs

Pain: ① ② ③ ④ ⑤		Stress: ① ② ③ ④ ⑤	
Nausea: ① ② ③ ④ ⑤		Anxiety: ① ② ③ ④ ⑤	
Inflammation: ① ② ③ ④ ⑤		Insomnia: ① ② ③ ④ ⑤	
Appetite: ① ② ③ ④ ⑤		Depression: ① ② ③ ④ ⑤	

Other positive effects: _____

Adverse effects

Anxiety: ① ② ③ ④ ⑤   Dry Mouth: ① ② ③ ④ ⑤

Munchies: ① ② ③ ④ ⑤   Fatigue: ① ② ③ ④ ⑤

Other adverse effects: _____

Notes

My Rating: 🍁 🍁 🍁 🍁 🍁

Strain:_____ Distributor:_____

PRICE: _____

TOTAL ACQUIRED: _____

PURCHASE DATE: _____

DISTRIBUTOR #: _____

description / notes

DOSAGE / INSTRUCTIONS	CERTIFICATE OF ANALYSIS	
	☐ Yes	☐ No

FORM
☐ Flower
☐ Edible
☐ Oil
☐ Tincture
☐ _____

METHOD
☐ Smoked
☐ Vaped
☐ Ingested
☐ Topical
☐ _____

CONTENT
_____% CBD
_____% THC
_____% _____
_____% _____
_____% _____

VARIETY
☐ Indica
☐ Sativa
☐ Hybrid

Dose: _____ Smell / Taste: _____

Time to take effect: _____ Effect duration: _____

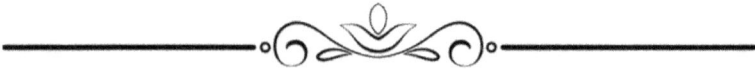

Reliefs

Pain: ① ② ③ ④ ⑤		Stress: ① ② ③ ④ ⑤		
Nausea: ① ② ③ ④ ⑤		Anxiety: ① ② ③ ④ ⑤		
Inflammation: ① ② ③ ④ ⑤		Insomnia: ① ② ③ ④ ⑤		
Appetite: ① ② ③ ④ ⑤		Depression: ① ② ③ ④ ⑤		

Other positive effects: _____

Adverse effects

Anxiety: ① ② ③ ④ ⑤	Dry Mouth: ① ② ③ ④ ⑤
Munchies: ① ② ③ ④ ⑤	Fatigue: ① ② ③ ④ ⑤

Other adverse effects: _____

Notes

My Rating: 🍁 🍁 🍁 🍁 🍁

DATE:	ENTRY:	22

Strain:_____ Distributor:_____

PRICE: _____

TOTAL ACQUIRED: _____

PURCHASE DATE: _____

DISTRIBUTOR #: _____

description / notes

DOSAGE / INSTRUCTIONS	CERTIFICATE OF ANALYSIS	
	☐ Yes	☐ No

FORM
☐ Flower
☐ Edible
☐ Oil
☐ Tincture
☐ _____

METHOD
☐ Smoked
☐ Vaped
☐ Ingested
☐ Topical
☐ _____

CONTENT
_____% CBD
_____% THC
_____% _____
_____% _____
_____% _____

VARIETY
☐ Indica
☐ Sativa
☐ Hybrid

Dose: _____ Smell / Taste: _____

Time to take effect: _____ Effect duration: _____

Reliefs

Pain:	1 2 3 4 5	Stress:	1 2 3 4 5
Nausea:	1 2 3 4 5	Anxiety:	1 2 3 4 5
Inflammation:	1 2 3 4 5	Insomnia:	1 2 3 4 5
Appetite:	1 2 3 4 5	Depression:	1 2 3 4 5

Other positive effects: _____

Adverse effects

Anxiety:	1 2 3 4 5	Dry Mouth:	1 2 3 4 5
Munchies:	1 2 3 4 5	Fatigue:	1 2 3 4 5

Other adverse effects: _____

Notes

My Rating: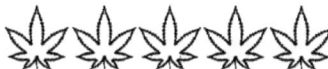

DATE:	ENTRY:	23

Strain:_____ Distributor:_____

PRICE: _____

TOTAL ACQUIRED: _____

PURCHASE DATE: _____

DISTRIBUTOR #: _____

description / notes

DOSAGE / INSTRUCTIONS	CERTIFICATE OF ANALYSIS	
	☐ Yes	☐ No

FORM
☐ Flower
☐ Edible
☐ Oil
☐ Tincture
☐ _____

METHOD
☐ Smoked
☐ Vaped
☐ Ingested
☐ Topical
☐ _____

CONTENT
_____% CBD
_____% THC
_____% _____
_____% _____
_____% _____

VARIETY
☐ Indica
☐ Sativa
☐ Hybrid

Dose: _____ Smell / Taste: _____

Time to take effect: _____ Effect duration: _____

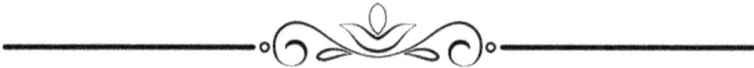

Reliefs

Pain:	①	②	③	④	⑤	Stress:	①	②	③	④ ⑤
Nausea:	①	②	③	④	⑤	Anxiety:	①	②	③	④ ⑤
Inflammation:	①	②	③	④	⑤	Insomnia:	①	②	③	④ ⑤
Appetite:	①	②	③	④	⑤	Depression:	①	②	③	④ ⑤

Other positive effects: _____

Adverse effects

Anxiety:	①	②	③	④	⑤	Dry Mouth:	①	②	③	④ ⑤
Munchies:	①	②	③	④	⑤	Fatigue:	①	②	③	④ ⑤

Other adverse effects: _____

Notes

My Rating: 🍁🍁🍁🍁🍁

DATE:	ENTRY:	24

Strain:_____ Distributor:_____

PRICE: _____	*description / notes*
TOTAL ACQUIRED: _____	
PURCHASE DATE: _____	
DISTRIBUTOR #: _____	

DOSAGE / INSTRUCTIONS	CERTIFICATE OF ANALYSIS	
	☐ Yes	☐ No

FORM	METHOD	CONTENT	VARIETY
☐ Flower	☐ Smoked	_____% CBD	☐ Indica
☐ Edible	☐ Vaped	_____% THC	☐ Sativa
☐ Oil	☐ Ingested	_____% _____	☐ Hybrid
☐ Tincture	☐ Topical	_____% _____	
☐ _____	☐ _____	_____% _____	

Dose: _____ Smell / Taste: _____

Time to take effect: _____ Effect duration: _____

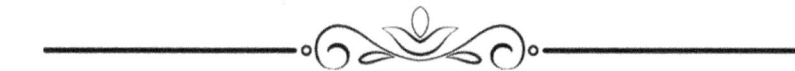

Reliefs

Pain:	① ② ③ ④ ⑤	Stress:	① ② ③ ④ ⑤
Nausea:	① ② ③ ④ ⑤	Anxiety:	① ② ③ ④ ⑤
Inflammation:	① ② ③ ④ ⑤	Insomnia:	① ② ③ ④ ⑤
Appetite:	① ② ③ ④ ⑤	Depression:	① ② ③ ④ ⑤

Other positive effects: _____

Adverse effects

Anxiety:	① ② ③ ④ ⑤	Dry Mouth:	① ② ③ ④ ⑤
Munchies:	① ② ③ ④ ⑤	Fatigue:	① ② ③ ④ ⑤

Other adverse effects: _____

Notes

My Rating: 🍁 🍁 🍁 🍁 🍁

Strain:_____ Distributor:_____

PRICE: _____

TOTAL ACQUIRED: _____

PURCHASE DATE: _____

DISTRIBUTOR #: _____

description / notes

DOSAGE / INSTRUCTIONS	CERTIFICATE OF ANALYSIS
	☐ Yes ☐ No

FORM
☐ Flower
☐ Edible
☐ Oil
☐ Tincture
☐ _____

METHOD
☐ Smoked
☐ Vaped
☐ Ingested
☐ Topical
☐ _____

CONTENT
_____% CBD
_____% THC
_____% _____
_____% _____
_____% _____

VARIETY
☐ Indica
☐ Sativa
☐ Hybrid

Dose: _____ Smell / Taste: _____

Time to take effect: _____ Effect duration: _____

Reliefs

Pain:	① ② ③ ④ ⑤	Stress:	① ② ③ ④ ⑤
Nausea:	① ② ③ ④ ⑤	Anxiety:	① ② ③ ④ ⑤
Inflammation:	① ② ③ ④ ⑤	Insomnia:	① ② ③ ④ ⑤
Appetite:	① ② ③ ④ ⑤	Depression:	① ② ③ ④ ⑤

Other positive effects: _____

Adverse effects

Anxiety:	① ② ③ ④ ⑤	Dry Mouth:	① ② ③ ④ ⑤
Munchies:	① ② ③ ④ ⑤	Fatigue:	① ② ③ ④ ⑤

Other adverse effects: _____

Notes

My Rating: 🍁 🍁 🍁 🍁 🍁

DATE: _____ ENTRY: 26

Strain:_____ Distributor:_____

PRICE: _____

TOTAL ACQUIRED: _____

PURCHASE DATE: _____

DISTRIBUTOR #: _____

description / notes

DOSAGE / INSTRUCTIONS	CERTIFICATE OF ANALYSIS	
	☐ Yes	☐ No

FORM
☐ Flower

☐ Edible

☐ Oil

☐ Tincture

☐ _____

METHOD
☐ Smoked

☐ Vaped

☐ Ingested

☐ Topical

☐ _____

CONTENT
_____% CBD

_____% THC

_____% _____

_____% _____

_____% _____

VARIETY
☐ Indica

☐ Sativa

☐ Hybrid

Dose: _____ Smell / Taste: _____

Time to take effect: _____ Effect duration: _____

Reliefs

Pain:	①	②	③	④	⑤	Stress:	①	②	③	④	⑤
Nausea:	①	②	③	④	⑤	Anxiety:	①	②	③	④	⑤
Inflammation:	①	②	③	④	⑤	Insomnia:	①	②	③	④	⑤
Appetite:	①	②	③	④	⑤	Depression:	①	②	③	④	⑤

Other positive effects: _____

Adverse effects

Anxiety:	①	②	③	④	⑤	Dry Mouth:	①	②	③	④	⑤
Munchies:	①	②	③	④	⑤	Fatigue:	①	②	③	④	⑤

Other adverse effects: _____

Notes

_____

_____

My Rating: 🍁 🍁 🍁 🍁 🍁

DATE:		ENTRY:	27

Strain:_____ Distributor:_____

PRICE: _____	description / notes
TOTAL ACQUIRED: _____	
PURCHASE DATE: _____	
DISTRIBUTOR #: _____	

DOSAGE / INSTRUCTIONS	CERTIFICATE OF ANALYSIS	
	☐ Yes	☐ No

FORM
- ☐ Flower
- ☐ Edible
- ☐ Oil
- ☐ Tincture
- ☐ _____

METHOD
- ☐ Smoked
- ☐ Vaped
- ☐ Ingested
- ☐ Topical
- ☐ _____

CONTENT
- _____% CBD
- _____% THC
- _____% _____
- _____% _____
- _____% _____

VARIETY
- ☐ Indica
- ☐ Sativa
- ☐ Hybrid

Dose: _____ Smell / Taste: _____

Time to take effect: _____ Effect duration: _____

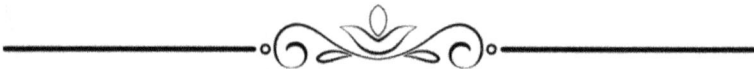

Reliefs

Pain:	①	②	③	④	⑤	Stress:	①	②	③	④ ⑤
Nausea:	①	②	③	④	⑤	Anxiety:	①	②	③	④ ⑤
Inflammation:	①	②	③	④	⑤	Insomnia:	①	②	③	④ ⑤
Appetite:	①	②	③	④	⑤	Depression:	①	②	③	④ ⑤

Other positive effects: _____

Adverse effects

Anxiety:	①	②	③	④	⑤	Dry Mouth:	①	②	③	④ ⑤
Munchies:	①	②	③	④	⑤	Fatigue:	①	②	③	④ ⑤

Other adverse effects: _____

Notes

My Rating: 🍁 🍁 🍁 🍁 🍁

DATE:	ENTRY:	28

Strain:_____ Distributor:_____

PRICE: _____	*description / notes*
TOTAL ACQUIRED: _____	
PURCHASE DATE: _____	
DISTRIBUTOR #: _____	

DOSAGE / INSTRUCTIONS	CERTIFICATE OF ANALYSIS	
	☐ Yes	☐ No

FORM	METHOD	CONTENT	VARIETY
☐ Flower	☐ Smoked	____% CBD	☐ Indica
☐ Edible	☐ Vaped	____% THC	☐ Sativa
☐ Oil	☐ Ingested	____% ____	☐ Hybrid
☐ Tincture	☐ Topical	____% ____	
☐ _____	☐ _____	____% ____	

Dose: _____ Smell / Taste: _____

Time to take effect: _____ Effect duration: _____

Reliefs

Pain:	① ② ③ ④ ⑤	Stress:	① ② ③ ④ ⑤
Nausea:	① ② ③ ④ ⑤	Anxiety:	① ② ③ ④ ⑤
Inflammation:	① ② ③ ④ ⑤	Insomnia:	① ② ③ ④ ⑤
Appetite:	① ② ③ ④ ⑤	Depression:	① ② ③ ④ ⑤

Other positive effects: _____

Adverse effects

Anxiety:	① ② ③ ④ ⑤	Dry Mouth:	① ② ③ ④ ⑤
Munchies:	① ② ③ ④ ⑤	Fatigue:	① ② ③ ④ ⑤

Other adverse effects: _____

Notes

_____

My Rating: 🍁 🍁 🍁 🍁 🍁

Strain:_____ Distributor:_____

PRICE: _____

TOTAL ACQUIRED: _____

PURCHASE DATE: _____

DISTRIBUTOR #: _____

description / notes

DOSAGE / INSTRUCTIONS	CERTIFICATE OF ANALYSIS	
	☐ Yes	☐ No

FORM
☐ Flower

☐ Edible

☐ Oil

☐ Tincture

☐ _____

METHOD
☐ Smoked

☐ Vaped

☐ Ingested

☐ Topical

☐ _____

CONTENT
_____% CBD

_____% THC

_____% _____

_____% _____

_____% _____

VARIETY
☐ Indica

☐ Sativa

☐ Hybrid

Dose: _____ Smell / Taste: _____

Time to take effect: _____ Effect duration: _____

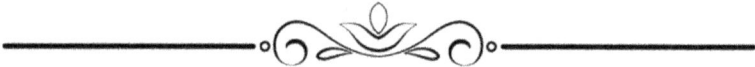

Reliefs

Pain:	①	②	③	④	⑤	Stress:	①	②	③	④	⑤
Nausea:	①	②	③	④	⑤	Anxiety:	①	②	③	④	⑤
Inflammation:	①	②	③	④	⑤	Insomnia:	①	②	③	④	⑤
Appetite:	①	②	③	④	⑤	Depression:	①	②	③	④	⑤

Other positive effects: _____

Adverse effects

Anxiety:	①	②	③	④	⑤	Dry Mouth:	①	②	③	④	⑤
Munchies:	①	②	③	④	⑤	Fatigue:	①	②	③	④	⑤

Other adverse effects: _____

Notes

My Rating: 🍁 🍁 🍁 🍁 🍁

Strain:_____ Distributor:_____

PRICE: _____
TOTAL ACQUIRED: _____
PURCHASE DATE: _____
DISTRIBUTOR #: _____

description / notes

DOSAGE / INSTRUCTIONS	CERTIFICATE OF ANALYSIS	
	☐ Yes	☐ No

FORM
☐ Flower
☐ Edible
☐ Oil
☐ Tincture
☐ _____

METHOD
☐ Smoked
☐ Vaped
☐ Ingested
☐ Topical
☐ _____

CONTENT
____% CBD
____% THC
____% _____
____% _____
____% _____

VARIETY
☐ Indica
☐ Sativa
☐ Hybrid

Dose: _____ Smell / Taste: _____

Time to take effect: _____ Effect duration: _____

Reliefs
Pain: ① ② ③ ④ ⑤   Stress: ① ② ③ ④ ⑤
Nausea: ① ② ③ ④ ⑤   Anxiety: ① ② ③ ④ ⑤
Inflammation: ① ② ③ ④ ⑤   Insomnia: ① ② ③ ④ ⑤
Appetite: ① ② ③ ④ ⑤   Depression: ① ② ③ ④ ⑤

Other positive effects: _____

Adverse effects
Anxiety: ① ② ③ ④ ⑤   Dry Mouth: ① ② ③ ④ ⑤
Munchies: ① ② ③ ④ ⑤   Fatigue: ① ② ③ ④ ⑤

Other adverse effects: _____

Notes
_____

My Rating: 🍁 🍁 🍁 🍁 🍁

DATE:		ENTRY:	31

Strain:_____ Distributor:_____

PRICE: _____

TOTAL ACQUIRED: _____

PURCHASE DATE: _____

DISTRIBUTOR #: _____

description / notes

DOSAGE / INSTRUCTIONS	CERTIFICATE OF ANALYSIS	
	☐ Yes	☐ No

FORM
☐ Flower
☐ Edible
☐ Oil
☐ Tincture
☐ _____

METHOD
☐ Smoked
☐ Vaped
☐ Ingested
☐ Topical
☐ _____

CONTENT
_____% CBD
_____% THC
_____% _____
_____% _____
_____% _____

VARIETY
☐ Indica
☐ Sativa
☐ Hybrid

Dose: _____   Smell / Taste: _____

Time to take effect: _____   Effect duration: _____

Reliefs

Pain:	① ② ③ ④ ⑤					Stress:	① ② ③ ④ ⑤				
Nausea:	① ② ③ ④ ⑤					Anxiety:	① ② ③ ④ ⑤				
Inflammation:	① ② ③ ④ ⑤					Depression:	① ② ③ ④ ⑤				
Appetite:	① ② ③ ④ ⑤					Insomnia:	① ② ③ ④ ⑤				

Other positive effects: _____

Adverse effects

Anxiety:	① ② ③ ④ ⑤					Dry Mouth:	① ② ③ ④ ⑤				
Munchies:	① ② ③ ④ ⑤					Fatigue:	① ② ③ ④ ⑤				

Other adverse effects: _____

Notes

My Rating:

DATE:	ENTRY:	32

Strain:_____ Distributor:_____

PRICE: _____
TOTAL ACQUIRED: _____
PURCHASE DATE: _____
DISTRIBUTOR #: _____

description / notes

DOSAGE / INSTRUCTIONS	CERTIFICATE OF ANALYSIS	
	☐ Yes	☐ No

FORM
☐ Flower
☐ Edible
☐ Oil
☐ Tincture
☐ _____

METHOD
☐ Smoked
☐ Vaped
☐ Ingested
☐ Topical
☐ _____

CONTENT
_____% CBD
_____% THC
_____% _____
_____% _____
_____% _____

VARIETY
☐ Indica
☐ Sativa
☐ Hybrid

Dose: _____ Smell / Taste: _____

Time to take effect: _____ Effect duration: _____

Reliefs

Pain:	①	②	③	④	⑤	Stress:	①	②	③	④	⑤
Nausea:	①	②	③	④	⑤	Anxiety:	①	②	③	④	⑤
Inflammation:	①	②	③	④	⑤	Insomnia:	①	②	③	④	⑤
Appetite:	①	②	③	④	⑤	Depression:	①	②	③	④	⑤

Other positive effects: _____

Adverse effects

Anxiety:	①	②	③	④	⑤	Dry Mouth:	①	②	③	④	⑤
Munchies:	①	②	③	④	⑤	Fatigue:	①	②	③	④	⑤

Other adverse effects: _____

Notes

My Rating: 🍁🍁🍁🍁🍁

DATE:		ENTRY:	33

Strain:_____ Distributor:_____

PRICE: _____

TOTAL ACQUIRED: _____

PURCHASE DATE: _____

DISTRIBUTOR #: _____

description / notes

DOSAGE / INSTRUCTIONS	CERTIFICATE OF ANALYSIS	
	☐ Yes	☐ No

FORM
☐ Flower
☐ Edible
☐ Oil
☐ Tincture
☐ _____

METHOD
☐ Smoked
☐ Vaped
☐ Ingested
☐ Topical
☐ _____

CONTENT
_____% CBD
_____% THC
_____% _____
_____% _____
_____% _____

VARIETY
☐ Indica
☐ Sativa
☐ Hybrid

Dose: _____ Smell / Taste: _____

Time to take effect: _____ Effect duration: _____

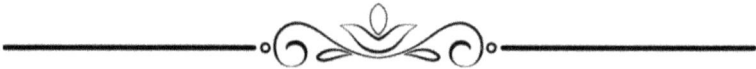

Reliefs

Pain:	① ② ③ ④ ⑤	Stress:	① ② ③ ④ ⑤
Nausea:	① ② ③ ④ ⑤	Anxiety:	① ② ③ ④ ⑤
Inflammation:	① ② ③ ④ ⑤	Insomnia:	① ② ③ ④ ⑤
Appetite:	① ② ③ ④ ⑤	Depression:	① ② ③ ④ ⑤

Other positive effects: _____

Adverse effects

Anxiety:	① ② ③ ④ ⑤	Dry Mouth:	① ② ③ ④ ⑤
Munchies:	① ② ③ ④ ⑤	Fatigue:	① ② ③ ④ ⑤

Other adverse effects: _____

Notes

My Rating: 🍁 🍁 🍁 🍁 🍁

Strain: _____ Distributor: _____

PRICE: _____

TOTAL ACQUIRED: _____

PURCHASE DATE: _____

DISTRIBUTOR #: _____

description / notes

DOSAGE / INSTRUCTIONS	CERTIFICATE OF ANALYSIS	
	☐ Yes	☐ No

FORM
☐ Flower
☐ Edible
☐ Oil
☐ Tincture
☐ _____

METHOD
☐ Smoked
☐ Vaped
☐ Ingested
☐ Topical
☐ _____

CONTENT
_____% CBD
_____% THC
_____% _____
_____% _____
_____% _____

VARIETY
☐ Indica
☐ Sativa
☐ Hybrid

Dose: _____   Smell / Taste: _____

Time to take effect: _____   Effect duration: _____

Reliefs

Pain: ① ② ③ ④ ⑤   Stress: ① ② ③ ④ ⑤

Nausea: ① ② ③ ④ ⑤   Anxiety: ① ② ③ ④ ⑤

Inflammation: ① ② ③ ④ ⑤   Insomnia: ① ② ③ ④ ⑤

Appetite: ① ② ③ ④ ⑤   Depression: ① ② ③ ④ ⑤

Other positive effects: _____

Adverse effects

Anxiety: ① ② ③ ④ ⑤   Dry Mouth: ① ② ③ ④ ⑤

Munchies: ① ② ③ ④ ⑤   Fatigue: ① ② ③ ④ ⑤

Other adverse effects: _____

Notes

My Rating: 🍁 🍁 🍁 🍁 🍁

DATE:		ENTRY:	35

Strain:_____ Distributor:_____

PRICE: _____
TOTAL ACQUIRED: _____
PURCHASE DATE: _____
DISTRIBUTOR #: _____

description / notes

DOSAGE / INSTRUCTIONS	CERTIFICATE OF ANALYSIS
	☐ Yes ☐ No

FORM
☐ Flower
☐ Edible
☐ Oil
☐ Tincture
☐ _____

METHOD
☐ Smoked
☐ Vaped
☐ Ingested
☐ Topical
☐ _____

CONTENT
_____% CBD
_____% THC
_____% _____
_____% _____
_____% _____

VARIETY
☐ Indica
☐ Sativa
☐ Hybrid

Dose: _____ Smell / Taste: _____

Time to take effect: _____ Effect duration: _____

Reliefs

Pain: 1 2 3 4 5   Stress: 1 2 3 4 5
Nausea: 1 2 3 4 5   Anxiety: 1 2 3 4 5
Inflammation: 1 2 3 4 5   Insomnia: 1 2 3 4 5
Appetite: 1 2 3 4 5   Depression: 1 2 3 4 5

Other positive effects: _____

Adverse effects

Anxiety: 1 2 3 4 5   Dry Mouth: 1 2 3 4 5
Munchies: 1 2 3 4 5   Fatigue: 1 2 3 4 5

Other adverse effects: _____

Notes

My Rating: ☆ ☆ ☆ ☆ ☆

Strain:_____ Distributor:_____

PRICE: _____

TOTAL ACQUIRED: _____

PURCHASE DATE: _____

DISTRIBUTOR #: _____

description / notes

DOSAGE / INSTRUCTIONS	CERTIFICATE OF ANALYSIS	
	☐ Yes	☐ No

FORM
☐ Flower
☐ Edible
☐ Oil
☐ Tincture
☐ _____

METHOD
☐ Smoked
☐ Vaped
☐ Ingested
☐ Topical
☐ _____

CONTENT
_____% CBD
_____% THC
_____% _____
_____% _____
_____% _____

VARIETY
☐ Indica
☐ Sativa
☐ Hybrid

Dose: _____ Smell / Taste: _____

Time to take effect: _____ Effect duration: _____

Reliefs

Pain: ① ② ③ ④ ⑤   Stress: ① ② ③ ④ ⑤

Nausea: ① ② ③ ④ ⑤   Anxiety: ① ② ③ ④ ⑤

Inflammation: ① ② ③ ④ ⑤   Insomnia: ① ② ③ ④ ⑤

Appetite: ① ② ③ ④ ⑤   Depression: ① ② ③ ④ ⑤

Other positive effects: _____

Adverse effects

Anxiety: ① ② ③ ④ ⑤   Dry Mouth: ① ② ③ ④ ⑤

Munchies: ① ② ③ ④ ⑤   Fatigue: ① ② ③ ④ ⑤

Other adverse effects: _____

Notes

My Rating: 🍁 🍁 🍁 🍁 🍁

DATE:		ENTRY:	37

Strain:_____ Distributor:_____

PRICE: _____	description / notes
TOTAL ACQUIRED: _____	
PURCHASE DATE: _____	
DISTRIBUTOR #: _____	

DOSAGE / INSTRUCTIONS	CERTIFICATE OF ANALYSIS	
	☐ Yes	☐ No

FORM	METHOD	CONTENT	VARIETY
☐ Flower	☐ Smoked	_____% CBD	☐ Indica
☐ Edible	☐ Vaped	_____% THC	☐ Sativa
☐ Oil	☐ Ingested	_____% _____	☐ Hybrid
☐ Tincture	☐ Topical	_____% _____	
☐ _____	☐ _____	_____% _____	

Dose: _____ Smell / Taste: _____

Time to take effect: _____ Effect duration: _____

Reliefs

Pain:	① ② ③ ④ ⑤	Stress:	① ② ③ ④ ⑤
Nausea:	① ② ③ ④ ⑤	Anxiety:	① ② ③ ④ ⑤
Inflammation:	① ② ③ ④ ⑤	Insomnia:	① ② ③ ④ ⑤
Appetite:	① ② ③ ④ ⑤	Depression:	① ② ③ ④ ⑤

Other positive effects: _____

Adverse effects

Anxiety:	① ② ③ ④ ⑤	Dry Mouth:	① ② ③ ④ ⑤
Munchies:	① ② ③ ④ ⑤	Fatigue:	① ② ③ ④ ⑤

Other adverse effects: _____

Notes

My Rating: 🍁 🍁 🍁 🍁 🍁

DATE:	ENTRY:	38

Strain:_____ Distributor:_____

PRICE: _____
TOTAL ACQUIRED: _____
PURCHASE DATE: _____
DISTRIBUTOR #: _____

description / notes

DOSAGE / INSTRUCTIONS	CERTIFICATE OF ANALYSIS	
	☐ Yes	☐ No

FORM
☐ Flower
☐ Edible
☐ Oil
☐ Tincture
☐ _____

METHOD
☐ Smoked
☐ Vaped
☐ Ingested
☐ Topical
☐ _____

CONTENT
_____% CBD
_____% THC
_____% _____
_____% _____
_____% _____

VARIETY
☐ Indica
☐ Sativa
☐ Hybrid

Dose: _____ Smell / Taste: _____

Time to take effect: _____ Effect duration: _____

Reliefs

Pain:	① ② ③ ④ ⑤	Stress:	① ② ③ ④ ⑤
Nausea:	① ② ③ ④ ⑤	Anxiety:	① ② ③ ④ ⑤
Inflammation:	① ② ③ ④ ⑤	Insomnia:	① ② ③ ④ ⑤
Appetite:	① ② ③ ④ ⑤	Depression:	① ② ③ ④ ⑤

Other positive effects: _____

Adverse effects

Anxiety:	① ② ③ ④ ⑤	Dry Mouth:	① ② ③ ④ ⑤
Munchies:	① ② ③ ④ ⑤	Fatigue:	① ② ③ ④ ⑤

Other adverse effects: _____

Notes

My Rating: 🍁 🍁 🍁 🍁 🍁

DATE:	ENTRY:	39

Strain:_____ Distributor:_____

PRICE: _____

TOTAL ACQUIRED: _____

PURCHASE DATE: _____

DISTRIBUTOR #: _____

description / notes

DOSAGE / INSTRUCTIONS	CERTIFICATE OF ANALYSIS	
	☐ Yes	☐ No

FORM
☐ Flower
☐ Edible
☐ Oil
☐ Tincture
☐ _____

METHOD
☐ Smoked
☐ Vaped
☐ Ingested
☐ Topical
☐ _____

CONTENT
_____% CBD
_____% THC
_____% _____
_____% _____
_____% _____

VARIETY
☐ Indica
☐ Sativa
☐ Hybrid

Dose: _____ Smell / Taste: _____

Time to take effect: _____ Effect duration: _____

Reliefs

Pain:	① ② ③ ④ ⑤	Stress:	① ② ③ ④ ⑤
Nausea:	① ② ③ ④ ⑤	Anxiety:	① ② ③ ④ ⑤
Inflammation:	① ② ③ ④ ⑤	Insomnia:	① ② ③ ④ ⑤
Appetite:	① ② ③ ④ ⑤	Depression:	① ② ③ ④ ⑤

Other positive effects: _____

Adverse effects

Anxiety:	① ② ③ ④ ⑤	Dry Mouth:	① ② ③ ④ ⑤
Munchies:	① ② ③ ④ ⑤	Fatigue:	① ② ③ ④ ⑤

Other adverse effects: _____

Notes

My Rating: 🍁 🍁 🍁 🍁 🍁

Strain:_____ Distributor:_____

PRICE: _____
TOTAL ACQUIRED: _____
PURCHASE DATE: _____
DISTRIBUTOR #: _____

description / notes

DOSAGE / INSTRUCTIONS	CERTIFICATE OF ANALYSIS	
	☐ Yes	☐ No

FORM
☐ Flower
☐ Edible
☐ Oil
☐ Tincture
☐ _____

METHOD
☐ Smoked
☐ Vaped
☐ Ingested
☐ Topical
☐ _____

CONTENT
_____% CBD
_____% THC
_____% _____
_____% _____
_____% _____

VARIETY
☐ Indica
☐ Sativa
☐ Hybrid

Dose: _____ Smell / Taste: _____

Time to take effect: _____ Effect duration: _____

Reliefs

Pain: ① ② ③ ④ ⑤   Stress: ① ② ③ ④ ⑤
Nausea: ① ② ③ ④ ⑤   Anxiety: ① ② ③ ④ ⑤
Inflammation: ① ② ③ ④ ⑤   Insomnia: ① ② ③ ④ ⑤
Appetite: ① ② ③ ④ ⑤   Depression: ① ② ③ ④ ⑤

Other positive effects: _____

Adverse effects

Anxiety: ① ② ③ ④ ⑤   Dry Mouth: ① ② ③ ④ ⑤
Munchies: ① ② ③ ④ ⑤   Fatigue: ① ② ③ ④ ⑤

Other adverse effects: _____

Notes

My Rating: ✿ ✿ ✿ ✿ ✿

DATE:		ENTRY:	41

Strain:_____ Distributor:_____

PRICE: _____

TOTAL ACQUIRED: _____

PURCHASE DATE: _____

DISTRIBUTOR #: _____

description / notes

DOSAGE / INSTRUCTIONS	CERTIFICATE OF ANALYSIS	
	☐ Yes	☐ No

FORM
☐ Flower
☐ Edible
☐ Oil
☐ Tincture
☐ _____

METHOD
☐ Smoked
☐ Vaped
☐ Ingested
☐ Topical
☐ _____

CONTENT
_____% CBD
_____% THC
_____% _____
_____% _____
_____% _____

VARIETY
☐ Indica
☐ Sativa
☐ Hybrid

Dose: _____ Smell / Taste: _____

Time to take effect: _____ Effect duration: _____

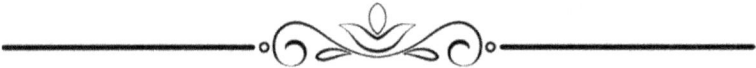

Reliefs

Pain:	① ② ③ ④ ⑤	Stress:	① ② ③ ④ ⑤
Nausea:	① ② ③ ④ ⑤	Anxiety:	① ② ③ ④ ⑤
Inflammation:	① ② ③ ④ ⑤	Insomnia:	① ② ③ ④ ⑤
Appetite:	① ② ③ ④ ⑤	Depression:	① ② ③ ④ ⑤

Other positive effects: _____

Adverse effects

Anxiety:	① ② ③ ④ ⑤	Dry Mouth:	① ② ③ ④ ⑤
Munchies:	① ② ③ ④ ⑤	Fatigue:	① ② ③ ④ ⑤

Other adverse effects: _____

Notes

My Rating: ✿ ✿ ✿ ✿ ✿

DATE:		ENTRY:	42

Strain:_____ Distributor:_____

PRICE: _____
TOTAL ACQUIRED: _____
PURCHASE DATE: _____
DISTRIBUTOR #: _____

description / notes

DOSAGE / INSTRUCTIONS	CERTIFICATE OF ANALYSIS	
	☐ Yes	☐ No

FORM
☐ Flower
☐ Edible
☐ Oil
☐ Tincture
☐ _____

METHOD
☐ Smoked
☐ Vaped
☐ Ingested
☐ Topical
☐ _____

CONTENT
_____% CBD
_____% THC
_____% _____
_____% _____
_____% _____

VARIETY
☐ Indica
☐ Sativa
☐ Hybrid

Dose: _____   Smell / Taste: _____

Time to take effect: _____   Effect duration: _____

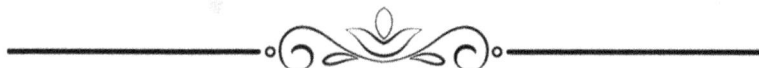

Reliefs

Pain:	①	②	③	④	⑤	Stress:	①	②	③	④	⑤
Nausea:	①	②	③	④	⑤	Anxiety:	①	②	③	④	⑤
Inflammation:	①	②	③	④	⑤	Insomnia:	①	②	③	④	⑤
Appetite:	①	②	③	④	⑤	Depression:	①	②	③	④	⑤

Other positive effects: _____

Adverse effects

Anxiety:	①	②	③	④	⑤	Dry Mouth:	①	②	③	④	⑤
Munchies:	①	②	③	④	⑤	Fatigue:	①	②	③	④	⑤

Other adverse effects: _____

Notes

My Rating:

Strain:_____ Distributor:_____

PRICE: _____

TOTAL ACQUIRED: _____

PURCHASE DATE: _____

DISTRIBUTOR #: _____

description / notes

DOSAGE / INSTRUCTIONS	CERTIFICATE OF ANALYSIS	
	☐ Yes	☐ No

FORM	METHOD	CONTENT	VARIETY
☐ Flower	☐ Smoked	_____% CBD	☐ Indica
☐ Edible	☐ Vaped	_____% THC	☐ Sativa
☐ Oil	☐ Ingested	_____% _____	☐ Hybrid
☐ Tincture	☐ Topical	_____% _____	
☐ _____	☐ _____	_____% _____	

Dose: _____ Smell / Taste: _____

Time to take effect: _____ Effect duration: _____

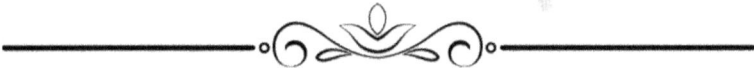

Reliefs

Pain:	① ② ③ ④ ⑤	Stress:	① ② ③ ④ ⑤
Nausea:	① ② ③ ④ ⑤	Anxiety:	① ② ③ ④ ⑤
Inflammation:	① ② ③ ④ ⑤	Insomnia:	① ② ③ ④ ⑤
Appetite:	① ② ③ ④ ⑤	Depression:	① ② ③ ④ ⑤

Other positive effects: _____

Adverse effects

Anxiety:	① ② ③ ④ ⑤	Dry Mouth:	① ② ③ ④ ⑤
Munchies:	① ② ③ ④ ⑤	Fatigue:	① ② ③ ④ ⑤

Other adverse effects: _____

Notes

My Rating:

Strain:_____ Distributor:_____

PRICE: _____

TOTAL ACQUIRED: _____

PURCHASE DATE: _____

DISTRIBUTOR #: _____

description / notes

DOSAGE / INSTRUCTIONS	CERTIFICATE OF ANALYSIS	
	☐ Yes	☐ No

FORM
☐ Flower
☐ Edible
☐ Oil
☐ Tincture
☐ _____

METHOD
☐ Smoked
☐ Vaped
☐ Ingested
☐ Topical
☐ _____

CONTENT
_____% CBD
_____% THC
_____% _____
_____% _____
_____% _____

VARIETY
☐ Indica
☐ Sativa
☐ Hybrid

Dose: _____ Smell / Taste: _____

Time to take effect: _____ Effect duration: _____

Reliefs

Pain: ① ② ③ ④ ⑤		Stress: ① ② ③ ④ ⑤	
Nausea: ① ② ③ ④ ⑤		Anxiety: ① ② ③ ④ ⑤	
Inflammation: ① ② ③ ④ ⑤		Insomnia: ① ② ③ ④ ⑤	
Appetite: ① ② ③ ④ ⑤		Depression: ① ② ③ ④ ⑤	

Other positive effects: _____

Adverse effects

Anxiety: ① ② ③ ④ ⑤	Dry Mouth: ① ② ③ ④ ⑤
Munchies: ① ② ③ ④ ⑤	Fatigue: ① ② ③ ④ ⑤

Other adverse effects: _____

Notes

My Rating: 🌿 🌿 🌿 🌿 🌿

DATE:	ENTRY:	45

Strain:_____ Distributor:_____

PRICE: _____
TOTAL ACQUIRED: _____
PURCHASE DATE: _____
DISTRIBUTOR #: _____

description / notes

DOSAGE / INSTRUCTIONS	CERTIFICATE OF ANALYSIS	
	☐ Yes	☐ No

FORM	METHOD	CONTENT	VARIETY
☐ Flower	☐ Smoked	_____% CBD	☐ Indica
☐ Edible	☐ Vaped	_____% THC	☐ Sativa
☐ Oil	☐ Ingested	_____% _____	☐ Hybrid
☐ Tincture	☐ Topical	_____% _____	
☐ _____	☐ _____	_____% _____	

Dose: _____ Smell / Taste: _____

Time to take effect: _____ Effect duration: _____

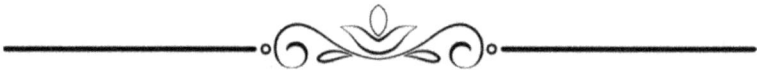

Reliefs

Pain: ① ② ③ ④ ⑤   Stress: ① ② ③ ④ ⑤
Nausea: ① ② ③ ④ ⑤   Anxiety: ① ② ③ ④ ⑤
Inflammation: ① ② ③ ④ ⑤   Insomnia: ① ② ③ ④ ⑤
Appetite: ① ② ③ ④ ⑤   Depression: ① ② ③ ④ ⑤

Other positive effects: _____

Adverse effects

Anxiety: ① ② ③ ④ ⑤   Dry Mouth: ① ② ③ ④ ⑤
Munchies: ① ② ③ ④ ⑤   Fatigue: ① ② ③ ④ ⑤

Other adverse effects: _____

Notes

My Rating: 🍁 🍁 🍁 🍁 🍁

Strain:_____ Distributor:_____

PRICE: _____
TOTAL ACQUIRED: _____
PURCHASE DATE: _____
DISTRIBUTOR #: _____

description / notes

DOSAGE / INSTRUCTIONS	CERTIFICATE OF ANALYSIS	
	☐ Yes	☐ No

FORM
☐ Flower
☐ Edible
☐ Oil
☐ Tincture
☐ _____

METHOD
☐ Smoked
☐ Vaped
☐ Ingested
☐ Topical
☐ _____

CONTENT
____% CBD
____% THC
____% _____
____% _____
____% _____

VARIETY
☐ Indica
☐ Sativa
☐ Hybrid

Dose: _____ Smell / Taste: _____

Time to take effect: _____ Effect duration: _____

Reliefs

Pain:	① ② ③ ④ ⑤					Stress:	① ② ③ ④ ⑤				
Nausea:	① ② ③ ④ ⑤					Anxiety:	① ② ③ ④ ⑤				
Inflammation:	① ② ③ ④ ⑤					Insomnia:	① ② ③ ④ ⑤				
Appetite:	① ② ③ ④ ⑤					Depression:	① ② ③ ④ ⑤				

Other positive effects: _____

Adverse effects

Anxiety: ① ② ③ ④ ⑤ Dry Mouth: ① ② ③ ④ ⑤
Munchies: ① ② ③ ④ ⑤ Fatigue: ① ② ③ ④ ⑤

Other adverse effects: _____

Notes

My Rating: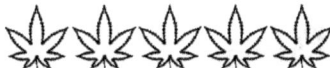

DATE:	ENTRY:	47

Strain:_____ Distributor:_____

PRICE: _____

TOTAL ACQUIRED: _____

PURCHASE DATE: _____

DISTRIBUTOR #: _____

description / notes

DOSAGE / INSTRUCTIONS	CERTIFICATE OF ANALYSIS	
	☐ Yes	☐ No

FORM
☐ Flower
☐ Edible
☐ Oil
☐ Tincture
☐ _____

METHOD
☐ Smoked
☐ Vaped
☐ Ingested
☐ Topical
☐ _____

CONTENT
_____% CBD
_____% THC
_____% _____
_____% _____
_____% _____

VARIETY
☐ Indica
☐ Sativa
☐ Hybrid

Dose: _____ Smell / Taste: _____

Time to take effect: _____ Effect duration: _____

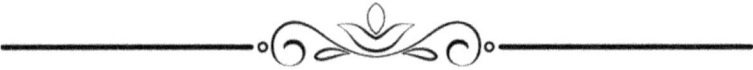

Reliefs

Pain:	① ② ③ ④ ⑤	Stress:	① ② ③ ④ ⑤
Nausea:	① ② ③ ④ ⑤	Anxiety:	① ② ③ ④ ⑤
Inflammation:	① ② ③ ④ ⑤	Insomnia:	① ② ③ ④ ⑤
Appetite:	① ② ③ ④ ⑤	Depression:	① ② ③ ④ ⑤

Other positive effects: _____

Adverse effects

Anxiety:	① ② ③ ④ ⑤	Dry Mouth:	① ② ③ ④ ⑤
Munchies:	① ② ③ ④ ⑤	Fatigue:	① ② ③ ④ ⑤

Other adverse effects: _____

Notes

My Rating:

Strain:_____ Distributor:_____

PRICE: _____

TOTAL ACQUIRED: _____

PURCHASE DATE: _____

DISTRIBUTOR #: _____

description / notes

DOSAGE / INSTRUCTIONS	CERTIFICATE OF ANALYSIS	
	☐ Yes	☐ No

FORM
☐ Flower
☐ Edible
☐ Oil
☐ Tincture
☐ _____

METHOD
☐ Smoked
☐ Vaped
☐ Ingested
☐ Topical
☐ _____

CONTENT
_____% CBD
_____% THC
_____% _____
_____% _____
_____% _____

VARIETY
☐ Indica
☐ Sativa
☐ Hybrid

Dose: _____ Smell / Taste: _____

Time to take effect: _____ Effect duration: _____

Reliefs

		Stress:	1 2 3 4 5
Pain:	1 2 3 4 5	Stress:	1 2 3 4 5
Nausea:	1 2 3 4 5	Anxiety:	1 2 3 4 5
Inflammation:	1 2 3 4 5	Insomnia:	1 2 3 4 5
Appetite:	1 2 3 4 5	Depression:	1 2 3 4 5

Other positive effects: _____

Adverse effects

Anxiety:	1 2 3 4 5	Dry Mouth:	1 2 3 4 5
Munchies:	1 2 3 4 5	Fatigue:	1 2 3 4 5

Other adverse effects: _____

Notes
_____

My Rating:

DATE:		ENTRY:	49

Strain:_____ Distributor:_____

PRICE: _____
TOTAL ACQUIRED: _____
PURCHASE DATE: _____
DISTRIBUTOR #: _____

description / notes

DOSAGE / INSTRUCTIONS	CERTIFICATE OF ANALYSIS	
	☐ Yes	☐ No

FORM
☐ Flower
☐ Edible
☐ Oil
☐ Tincture
☐ _____

METHOD
☐ Smoked
☐ Vaped
☐ Ingested
☐ Topical
☐ _____

CONTENT
_____% CBD
_____% THC
_____% _____
_____% _____
_____% _____

VARIETY
☐ Indica
☐ Sativa
☐ Hybrid

Dose: _____   Smell / Taste: _____

Time to take effect: _____   Effect duration: _____

Reliefs

Pain:	① ② ③ ④ ⑤		Stress:	① ② ③ ④ ⑤
Nausea:	① ② ③ ④ ⑤		Anxiety:	① ② ③ ④ ⑤
Inflammation:	① ② ③ ④ ⑤		Insomnia:	① ② ③ ④ ⑤
Appetite:	① ② ③ ④ ⑤		Depression:	① ② ③ ④ ⑤

Other positive effects: _____

Adverse effects

Anxiety:	① ② ③ ④ ⑤		Dry Mouth:	① ② ③ ④ ⑤
Munchies:	① ② ③ ④ ⑤		Fatigue:	① ② ③ ④ ⑤

Other adverse effects: _____

Notes

My Rating: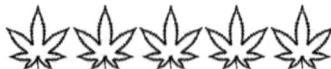

Strain:_____ Distributor:_____

PRICE:
TOTAL ACQUIRED:
PURCHASE DATE:
DISTRIBUTOR #:

description / notes

DOSAGE / INSTRUCTIONS	CERTIFICATE OF ANALYSIS	
	☐ Yes	☐ No

FORM
☐ Flower
☐ Edible
☐ Oil
☐ Tincture
☐ _____

METHOD
☐ Smoked
☐ Vaped
☐ Ingested
☐ Topical
☐ _____

CONTENT
_____% CBD
_____% THC
_____% _____
_____% _____
_____% _____

VARIETY
☐ Indica
☐ Sativa
☐ Hybrid

Dose: _____ Smell / Taste: _____

Time to take effect: _____ Effect duration: _____

Reliefs

Pain:	1	2	3	4	5	Stress:	1	2	3	4	5
Nausea:	1	2	3	4	5	Anxiety:	1	2	3	4	5
Inflammation:	1	2	3	4	5	Insomnia:	1	2	3	4	5
Appetite:	1	2	3	4	5	Depression:	1	2	3	4	5

Other positive effects: _____

Adverse effects

Anxiety:	1	2	3	4	5	Dry Mouth:	1	2	3	4	5
Munchies:	1	2	3	4	5	Fatigue:	1	2	3	4	5

Other adverse effects: _____

Notes

My Rating:

Strain:_____ Distributor:_____

PRICE: _____

TOTAL ACQUIRED: _____

PURCHASE DATE: _____

DISTRIBUTOR #: _____

description / notes

DOSAGE / INSTRUCTIONS	CERTIFICATE OF ANALYSIS	
	☐ Yes	☐ No

FORM
☐ Flower
☐ Edible
☐ Oil
☐ Tincture
☐ _____

METHOD
☐ Smoked
☐ Vaped
☐ Ingested
☐ Topical
☐ _____

CONTENT
_____% CBD
_____% THC
_____% _____
_____% _____
_____% _____

VARIETY
☐ Indica
☐ Sativa
☐ Hybrid

Dose: _____   Smell / Taste: _____

Time to take effect: _____   Effect duration: _____

Reliefs

Pain: ① ② ③ ④ ⑤		Stress: ① ② ③ ④ ⑤	
Nausea: ① ② ③ ④ ⑤		Anxiety: ① ② ③ ④ ⑤	
Inflammation: ① ② ③ ④ ⑤		Insomnia: ① ② ③ ④ ⑤	
Appetite: ① ② ③ ④ ⑤		Depression: ① ② ③ ④ ⑤	

Other positive effects: _____

Adverse effects

Anxiety: ① ② ③ ④ ⑤   Dry Mouth: ① ② ③ ④ ⑤

Munchies: ① ② ③ ④ ⑤   Fatigue: ① ② ③ ④ ⑤

Other adverse effects: _____

Notes

My Rating: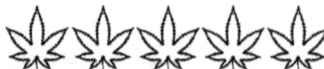

DATE: _____ ENTRY: **52**

Strain:_____ Distributor:_____

PRICE: _____
TOTAL ACQUIRED: _____
PURCHASE DATE: _____
DISTRIBUTOR #: _____

description / notes

DOSAGE / INSTRUCTIONS	CERTIFICATE OF ANALYSIS	
	☐ Yes	☐ No

FORM
☐ Flower
☐ Edible
☐ Oil
☐ Tincture
☐ _____

METHOD
☐ Smoked
☐ Vaped
☐ Ingested
☐ Topical
☐ _____

CONTENT
____% CBD
____% THC
____% ____
____% ____
____% ____

VARIETY
☐ Indica
☐ Sativa
☐ Hybrid

Dose: _____   Smell / Taste: _____

Time to take effect: _____   Effect duration: _____

Reliefs

Pain:	① ② ③ ④ ⑤	Stress:	① ② ③ ④ ⑤
Nausea:	① ② ③ ④ ⑤	Anxiety:	① ② ③ ④ ⑤
Inflammation:	① ② ③ ④ ⑤	Insomnia:	① ② ③ ④ ⑤
Appetite:	① ② ③ ④ ⑤	Depression:	① ② ③ ④ ⑤

Other positive effects: _____

Adverse effects

Anxiety:	① ② ③ ④ ⑤	Dry Mouth:	① ② ③ ④ ⑤
Munchies:	① ② ③ ④ ⑤	Fatigue:	① ② ③ ④ ⑤

Other adverse effects: _____

Notes
_____

My Rating: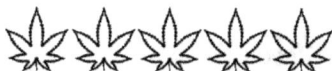

DATE:	ENTRY:	53

Strain:_____ Distributor:_____

PRICE: _____

TOTAL ACQUIRED: _____

PURCHASE DATE: _____

DISTRIBUTOR #: _____

description / notes

DOSAGE / INSTRUCTIONS	CERTIFICATE OF ANALYSIS	
	☐ Yes	☐ No

FORM	METHOD	CONTENT	VARIETY
☐ Flower	☐ Smoked	_____% CBD	☐ Indica
☐ Edible	☐ Vaped	_____% THC	☐ Sativa
☐ Oil	☐ Ingested	_____% _____	☐ Hybrid
☐ Tincture	☐ Topical	_____% _____	
☐ _____	☐ _____	_____% _____	

Dose: _____ Smell / Taste: _____

Time to take effect: _____ Effect duration: _____

Reliefs

Pain:	① ② ③ ④ ⑤	Stress:	① ② ③ ④ ⑤
Nausea:	① ② ③ ④ ⑤	Anxiety:	① ② ③ ④ ⑤
Inflammation:	① ② ③ ④ ⑤	Insomnia:	① ② ③ ④ ⑤
Appetite:	① ② ③ ④ ⑤	Depression:	① ② ③ ④ ⑤

Other positive effects: _____

Adverse effects

Anxiety:	① ② ③ ④ ⑤	Dry Mouth:	① ② ③ ④ ⑤
Munchies:	① ② ③ ④ ⑤	Fatigue:	① ② ③ ④ ⑤

Other adverse effects: _____

Notes
_____

My Rating:

DATE:	ENTRY:	54

Strain:_____ Distributor:_____

PRICE: _____

TOTAL ACQUIRED: _____

PURCHASE DATE: _____

DISTRIBUTOR #: _____

description / notes

DOSAGE / INSTRUCTIONS	CERTIFICATE OF ANALYSIS	
	☐ Yes	☐ No

FORM
☐ Flower
☐ Edible
☐ Oil
☐ Tincture
☐ _____

METHOD
☐ Smoked
☐ Vaped
☐ Ingested
☐ Topical
☐ _____

CONTENT
_____% CBD
_____% THC
_____% _____
_____% _____
_____% _____

VARIETY
☐ Indica
☐ Sativa
☐ Hybrid

Dose: _____ Smell / Taste: _____

Time to take effect: _____ Effect duration: _____

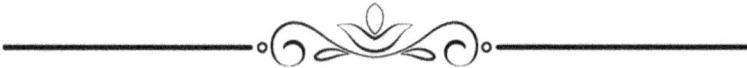

Reliefs

Pain: ① ② ③ ④ ⑤ Stress: ① ② ③ ④ ⑤

Nausea: ① ② ③ ④ ⑤ Anxiety: ① ② ③ ④ ⑤

Inflammation: ① ② ③ ④ ⑤ Insomnia: ① ② ③ ④ ⑤

Appetite: ① ② ③ ④ ⑤ Depression: ① ② ③ ④ ⑤

Other positive effects: _____

Adverse effects

Anxiety: ① ② ③ ④ ⑤ Dry Mouth: ① ② ③ ④ ⑤

Munchies: ① ② ③ ④ ⑤ Fatigue: ① ② ③ ④ ⑤

Other adverse effects: _____

Notes

_____

_____

My Rating: ✿ ✿ ✿ ✿ ✿

DATE:		ENTRY:	55

Strain:_____ Distributor:_____

PRICE: _____

TOTAL ACQUIRED: _____

PURCHASE DATE: _____

DISTRIBUTOR #: _____

description / notes

DOSAGE / INSTRUCTIONS	CERTIFICATE OF ANALYSIS	
	☐ Yes	☐ No

FORM
☐ Flower
☐ Edible
☐ Oil
☐ Tincture
☐ _____

METHOD
☐ Smoked
☐ Vaped
☐ Ingested
☐ Topical
☐ _____

CONTENT
_____% CBD
_____% THC
_____% _____
_____% _____
_____% _____

VARIETY
☐ Indica
☐ Sativa
☐ Hybrid

Dose: _____   Smell / Taste: _____

Time to take effect: _____   Effect duration: _____

Reliefs

Pain:	①	②	③	④	⑤	Stress:	①	②	③	④ ⑤
Nausea:	①	②	③	④	⑤	Anxiety:	①	②	③	④ ⑤
Inflammation:	①	②	③	④	⑤	Insomnia:	①	②	③	④ ⑤
Appetite:	①	②	③	④	⑤	Depression:	①	②	③	④ ⑤

Other positive effects: _____

Adverse effects

Anxiety:	①	②	③	④	⑤	Dry Mouth:	①	②	③	④ ⑤
Munchies:	①	②	③	④	⑤	Fatigue:	①	②	③	④ ⑤

Other adverse effects: _____

Notes

My Rating:

Strain:_____ Distributor:_____

PRICE: _____
TOTAL ACQUIRED: _____
PURCHASE DATE: _____
DISTRIBUTOR #: _____

description / notes

DOSAGE / INSTRUCTIONS	CERTIFICATE OF ANALYSIS	
	☐ Yes	☐ No

FORM	METHOD	CONTENT	VARIETY
☐ Flower	☐ Smoked	_____% CBD	☐ Indica
☐ Edible	☐ Vaped	_____% THC	☐ Sativa
☐ Oil	☐ Ingested	_____% _____	☐ Hybrid
☐ Tincture	☐ Topical	_____% _____	
☐ _____	☐ _____	_____% _____	

Dose: _____ Smell / Taste: _____

Time to take effect: _____ Effect duration: _____

Reliefs

Pain: ① ② ③ ④ ⑤   Stress: ① ② ③ ④ ⑤
Nausea: ① ② ③ ④ ⑤   Anxiety: ① ② ③ ④ ⑤
Inflammation: ① ② ③ ④ ⑤   Insomnia: ① ② ③ ④ ⑤
Appetite: ① ② ③ ④ ⑤   Depression: ① ② ③ ④ ⑤

Other positive effects: _____

Adverse effects

Anxiety: ① ② ③ ④ ⑤   Dry Mouth: ① ② ③ ④ ⑤
Munchies: ① ② ③ ④ ⑤   Fatigue: ① ② ③ ④ ⑤

Other adverse effects: _____

Notes

My Rating: 🌿 🌿 🌿 🌿 🌿

DATE:	ENTRY:	57

Strain:_____ Distributor:_____

PRICE: _____

TOTAL ACQUIRED: _____

PURCHASE DATE: _____

DISTRIBUTOR #: _____

description / notes

DOSAGE / INSTRUCTIONS	CERTIFICATE OF ANALYSIS	
	☐ Yes	☐ No

FORM
☐ Flower
☐ Edible
☐ Oil
☐ Tincture
☐ _____

METHOD
☐ Smoked
☐ Vaped
☐ Ingested
☐ Topical
☐ _____

CONTENT
_____% CBD
_____% THC
_____% _____
_____% _____
_____% _____

VARIETY
☐ Indica
☐ Sativa
☐ Hybrid

Dose: _____ Smell / Taste: _____

Time to take effect: _____ Effect duration: _____

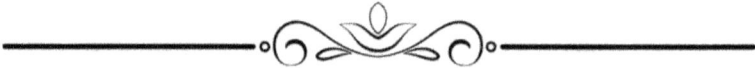

Reliefs

Pain:	① ② ③ ④ ⑤	Stress:	① ② ③ ④ ⑤
Nausea:	① ② ③ ④ ⑤	Anxiety:	① ② ③ ④ ⑤
Inflammation:	① ② ③ ④ ⑤	Insomnia:	① ② ③ ④ ⑤
Appetite:	① ② ③ ④ ⑤	Depression:	① ② ③ ④ ⑤

Other positive effects: _____

Adverse effects

Anxiety:	① ② ③ ④ ⑤	Dry Mouth:	① ② ③ ④ ⑤
Munchies:	① ② ③ ④ ⑤	Fatigue:	① ② ③ ④ ⑤

Other adverse effects: _____

Notes

My Rating: 🍁 🍁 🍁 🍁 🍁

DATE:		ENTRY:	58

Strain:_____ Distributor:_____

PRICE: _____

TOTAL ACQUIRED: _____

PURCHASE DATE: _____

DISTRIBUTOR #: _____

description / notes

DOSAGE / INSTRUCTIONS	CERTIFICATE OF ANALYSIS	
	☐ Yes	☐ No

FORM
☐ Flower
☐ Edible
☐ Oil
☐ Tincture
☐ _____

METHOD
☐ Smoked
☐ Vaped
☐ Ingested
☐ Topical
☐ _____

CONTENT
_____% CBD
_____% THC
_____% _____
_____% _____
_____% _____

VARIETY
☐ Indica
☐ Sativa
☐ Hybrid

Dose: _____ Smell / Taste: _____

Time to take effect: _____ Effect duration: _____

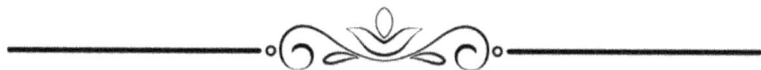

Reliefs

Pain:	① ② ③ ④ ⑤	Stress:	① ② ③ ④ ⑤
Nausea:	① ② ③ ④ ⑤	Anxiety:	① ② ③ ④ ⑤
Inflammation:	① ② ③ ④ ⑤	Insomnia:	① ② ③ ④ ⑤
Appetite:	① ② ③ ④ ⑤	Depression:	① ② ③ ④ ⑤

Other positive effects: _____

Adverse effects

Anxiety:	① ② ③ ④ ⑤	Dry Mouth:	① ② ③ ④ ⑤
Munchies:	① ② ③ ④ ⑤	Fatigue:	① ② ③ ④ ⑤

Other adverse effects: _____

Notes

My Rating: 🍁 🍁 🍁 🍁 🍁

DATE:	ENTRY:	59

Strain:_____ Distributor:_____

PRICE: _____	*description / notes*
TOTAL ACQUIRED: _____	
PURCHASE DATE: _____	
DISTRIBUTOR #: _____	

DOSAGE / INSTRUCTIONS	CERTIFICATE OF ANALYSIS	
	☐ Yes	☐ No

FORM	METHOD	CONTENT	VARIETY
☐ Flower	☐ Smoked	_____% CBD	☐ Indica
☐ Edible	☐ Vaped	_____% THC	☐ Sativa
☐ Oil	☐ Ingested	_____% _____	☐ Hybrid
☐ Tincture	☐ Topical	_____% _____	
☐ _____	☐ _____	_____% _____	

Dose: _____   Smell / Taste: _____

Time to take effect: _____   Effect duration: _____

Reliefs

Pain:	① ② ③ ④ ⑤	Stress:	① ② ③ ④ ⑤
Nausea:	① ② ③ ④ ⑤	Anxiety:	① ② ③ ④ ⑤
Inflammation:	① ② ③ ④ ⑤	Insomnia:	① ② ③ ④ ⑤
Appetite:	① ② ③ ④ ⑤	Depression:	① ② ③ ④ ⑤

Other positive effects: _____

Adverse effects

Anxiety:	① ② ③ ④ ⑤	Dry Mouth:	① ② ③ ④ ⑤
Munchies:	① ② ③ ④ ⑤	Fatigue:	① ② ③ ④ ⑤

Other adverse effects: _____

Notes

_____

My Rating: 🍁 🍁 🍁 🍁 🍁

Strain:_____ Distributor:_____

PRICE: _____

TOTAL ACQUIRED: _____

PURCHASE DATE: _____

DISTRIBUTOR #: _____

description / notes

DOSAGE / INSTRUCTIONS	CERTIFICATE OF ANALYSIS	
	☐ Yes	☐ No

FORM
☐ Flower
☐ Edible
☐ Oil
☐ Tincture
☐ _____

METHOD
☐ Smoked
☐ Vaped
☐ Ingested
☐ Topical
☐ _____

CONTENT
_____% CBD
_____% THC
_____% _____
_____% _____
_____% _____

VARIETY
☐ Indica
☐ Sativa
☐ Hybrid

Dose: _____ Smell / Taste: _____

Time to take effect: _____ Effect duration: _____

Reliefs

Pain: ① ② ③ ④ ⑤   Stress: ① ② ③ ④ ⑤

Nausea: ① ② ③ ④ ⑤   Anxiety: ① ② ③ ④ ⑤

Inflammation: ① ② ③ ④ ⑤   Insomnia: ① ② ③ ④ ⑤

Appetite: ① ② ③ ④ ⑤   Depression: ① ② ③ ④ ⑤

Other positive effects: _____

Adverse effects

Anxiety: ① ② ③ ④ ⑤   Dry Mouth: ① ② ③ ④ ⑤

Munchies: ① ② ③ ④ ⑤   Fatigue: ① ② ③ ④ ⑤

Other adverse effects: _____

Notes

_____

My Rating: 🌿 🌿 🌿 🌿 🌿

Strain:_____ Distributor:_____

PRICE: _____

TOTAL ACQUIRED: _____

PURCHASE DATE: _____

DISTRIBUTOR #: _____

description / notes

DOSAGE / INSTRUCTIONS	CERTIFICATE OF ANALYSIS	
	☐ Yes	☐ No

FORM
- ☐ Flower
- ☐ Edible
- ☐ Oil
- ☐ Tincture
- ☐ _____

METHOD
- ☐ Smoked
- ☐ Vaped
- ☐ Ingested
- ☐ Topical
- ☐ _____

CONTENT
- _____% CBD
- _____% THC
- _____% _____
- _____% _____
- _____% _____

VARIETY
- ☐ Indica
- ☐ Sativa
- ☐ Hybrid

Dose: _____ Smell / Taste: _____

Time to take effect: _____ Effect duration: _____

Reliefs

Pain: ① ② ③ ④ ⑤   Stress: ① ② ③ ④ ⑤

Nausea: ① ② ③ ④ ⑤   Anxiety: ① ② ③ ④ ⑤

Inflammation: ① ② ③ ④ ⑤   Depression: ① ② ③ ④ ⑤

Appetite: ① ② ③ ④ ⑤   Insomnia: ① ② ③ ④ ⑤

Other positive effects: _____

Adverse effects

Anxiety: ① ② ③ ④ ⑤   Dry Mouth: ① ② ③ ④ ⑤

Munchies: ① ② ③ ④ ⑤   Fatigue: ① ② ③ ④ ⑤

Other adverse effects: _____

Notes

My Rating: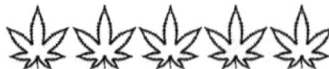

DATE: _____ ENTRY: 62

Strain:_____ Distributor:_____

PRICE: _____
TOTAL ACQUIRED: _____
PURCHASE DATE: _____
DISTRIBUTOR #: _____

description / notes

DOSAGE / INSTRUCTIONS	CERTIFICATE OF ANALYSIS	
	☐ Yes	☐ No

FORM
☐ Flower
☐ Edible
☐ Oil
☐ Tincture
☐ _____

METHOD
☐ Smoked
☐ Vaped
☐ Ingested
☐ Topical
☐ _____

CONTENT
_____% CBD
_____% THC
_____% _____
_____% _____
_____% _____

VARIETY
☐ Indica
☐ Sativa
☐ Hybrid

Dose: _____   Smell / Taste: _____

Time to take effect: _____   Effect duration: _____

Reliefs

Pain:	①②③④⑤	Stress:	①②③④⑤
Nausea:	①②③④⑤	Anxiety:	①②③④⑤
Inflammation:	①②③④⑤	Insomnia:	①②③④⑤
Appetite:	①②③④⑤	Depression:	①②③④⑤

Other positive effects: _____

Adverse effects

Anxiety:	①②③④⑤	Dry Mouth:	①②③④⑤
Munchies:	①②③④⑤	Fatigue:	①②③④⑤

Other adverse effects: _____

Notes
_____

My Rating: 🍁🍁🍁🍁🍁

Strain:_____ Distributor:_____

PRICE: _____
TOTAL ACQUIRED: _____
PURCHASE DATE: _____
DISTRIBUTOR #: _____

description / notes

DOSAGE / INSTRUCTIONS	CERTIFICATE OF ANALYSIS	
	☐ Yes	☐ No

FORM
☐ Flower
☐ Edible
☐ Oil
☐ Tincture
☐ _____

METHOD
☐ Smoked
☐ Vaped
☐ Ingested
☐ Topical
☐ _____

CONTENT
_____% CBD
_____% THC
_____% _____
_____% _____
_____% _____

VARIETY
☐ Indica
☐ Sativa
☐ Hybrid

Dose: _____ Smell / Taste: _____

Time to take effect: _____ Effect duration: _____

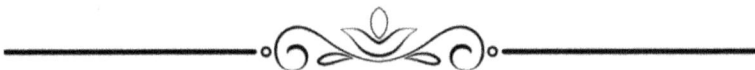

Reliefs

Pain:	① ② ③ ④ ⑤	Stress:	① ② ③ ④ ⑤
Nausea:	① ② ③ ④ ⑤	Anxiety:	① ② ③ ④ ⑤
Inflammation:	① ② ③ ④ ⑤	Insomnia:	① ② ③ ④ ⑤
Appetite:	① ② ③ ④ ⑤	Depression:	① ② ③ ④ ⑤

Other positive effects: _____

Adverse effects

Anxiety:	① ② ③ ④ ⑤	Dry Mouth:	① ② ③ ④ ⑤
Munchies:	① ② ③ ④ ⑤	Fatigue:	① ② ③ ④ ⑤

Other adverse effects: _____

Notes

My Rating: 🍁 🍁 🍁 🍁 🍁

DATE:	ENTRY:	64

Strain:_____ **Distributor:**_____

PRICE:	_____
TOTAL ACQUIRED:	_____
PURCHASE DATE:	_____
DISTRIBUTOR #:	_____

description / notes

DOSAGE / INSTRUCTIONS	CERTIFICATE OF ANALYSIS	
	☐ Yes	☐ No

FORM
☐ Flower
☐ Edible
☐ Oil
☐ Tincture
☐ _____

METHOD
☐ Smoked
☐ Vaped
☐ Ingested
☐ Topical
☐ _____

CONTENT
_____% CBD
_____% THC
_____% _____
_____% _____
_____% _____

VARIETY
☐ Indica
☐ Sativa
☐ Hybrid

Dose: _____   Smell / Taste: _____

Time to take effect: _____   Effect duration: _____

Reliefs

Pain:	① ② ③ ④ ⑤	Stress:	① ② ③ ④ ⑤
Nausea:	① ② ③ ④ ⑤	Anxiety:	① ② ③ ④ ⑤
Inflammation:	① ② ③ ④ ⑤	Insomnia:	① ② ③ ④ ⑤
Appetite:	① ② ③ ④ ⑤	Depression:	① ② ③ ④ ⑤

Other positive effects: _____

Adverse effects

Anxiety:	① ② ③ ④ ⑤	Dry Mouth:	① ② ③ ④ ⑤
Munchies:	① ② ③ ④ ⑤	Fatigue:	① ② ③ ④ ⑤

Other adverse effects: _____

Notes
_____

My Rating: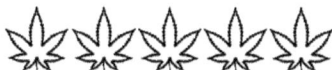

Strain:_____ Distributor:_____

PRICE: _____

TOTAL ACQUIRED: _____

PURCHASE DATE: _____

DISTRIBUTOR #: _____

description / notes

DOSAGE / INSTRUCTIONS	CERTIFICATE OF ANALYSIS	
	☐ Yes	☐ No

FORM
☐ Flower
☐ Edible
☐ Oil
☐ Tincture
☐ _____

METHOD
☐ Smoked
☐ Vaped
☐ Ingested
☐ Topical
☐ _____

CONTENT
_____% CBD
_____% THC
_____% _____
_____% _____
_____% _____

VARIETY
☐ Indica
☐ Sativa
☐ Hybrid

Dose: _____ Smell / Taste: _____

Time to take effect: _____ Effect duration: _____

Reliefs

Pain:	1	2	3	4	5	Stress:	1	2	3	4	5
Nausea:	1	2	3	4	5	Anxiety:	1	2	3	4	5
Inflammation:	1	2	3	4	5	Insomnia:	1	2	3	4	5
Appetite:	1	2	3	4	5	Depression:	1	2	3	4	5

Other positive effects: _____

Adverse effects

Anxiety:	1	2	3	4	5	Dry Mouth:	1	2	3	4	5
Munchies:	1	2	3	4	5	Fatigue:	1	2	3	4	5

Other adverse effects: _____

Notes

_____

My Rating:

DATE:	ENTRY:	66

Strain:_____ Distributor:_____

PRICE: _____
TOTAL ACQUIRED: _____
PURCHASE DATE: _____
DISTRIBUTOR #: _____

description / notes

DOSAGE / INSTRUCTIONS	CERTIFICATE OF ANALYSIS	
	☐ Yes	☐ No

FORM
☐ Flower
☐ Edible
☐ Oil
☐ Tincture
☐ _____

METHOD
☐ Smoked
☐ Vaped
☐ Ingested
☐ Topical
☐ _____

CONTENT
_____% CBD
_____% THC
_____% _____
_____% _____
_____% _____

VARIETY
☐ Indica
☐ Sativa
☐ Hybrid

Dose: _____ Smell / Taste: _____

Time to take effect: _____ Effect duration: _____

Reliefs

Pain:	1	2	3	4	5	Stress:	1	2	3	4	5
Nausea:	1	2	3	4	5	Anxiety:	1	2	3	4	5
Inflammation:	1	2	3	4	5	Insomnia:	1	2	3	4	5
Appetite:	1	2	3	4	5	Depression:	1	2	3	4	5

Other positive effects: _____

Adverse effects

Anxiety:	1	2	3	4	5	Dry Mouth:	1	2	3	4	5
Munchies:	1	2	3	4	5	Fatigue:	1	2	3	4	5

Other adverse effects: _____

Notes

My Rating:

Strain:_____ Distributor:_____

PRICE: _____
TOTAL ACQUIRED: _____
PURCHASE DATE: _____
DISTRIBUTOR #: _____

description / notes

DOSAGE / INSTRUCTIONS	CERTIFICATE OF ANALYSIS
	☐ Yes ☐ No

FORM	METHOD	CONTENT	VARIETY
☐ Flower	☐ Smoked	_____% CBD	☐ Indica
☐ Edible	☐ Vaped	_____% THC	☐ Sativa
☐ Oil	☐ Ingested	_____% _____	☐ Hybrid
☐ Tincture	☐ Topical	_____% _____	
☐ _____	☐ _____	_____% _____	

Dose: _____   Smell / Taste: _____

Time to take effect: _____   Effect duration: _____

Reliefs

Pain: ① ② ③ ④ ⑤   Stress: ① ② ③ ④ ⑤
Nausea: ① ② ③ ④ ⑤   Anxiety: ① ② ③ ④ ⑤
Inflammation: ① ② ③ ④ ⑤   Insomnia: ① ② ③ ④ ⑤
Appetite: ① ② ③ ④ ⑤   Depression: ① ② ③ ④ ⑤

Other positive effects: _____

Adverse effects

Anxiety: ① ② ③ ④ ⑤   Dry Mouth: ① ② ③ ④ ⑤
Munchies: ① ② ③ ④ ⑤   Fatigue: ① ② ③ ④ ⑤

Other adverse effects: _____

Notes

My Rating: 🍁 🍁 🍁 🍁 🍁

Strain:_____ **Distributor:**_____

PRICE: _____
TOTAL ACQUIRED: _____
PURCHASE DATE: _____
DISTRIBUTOR #: _____

description / notes

DOSAGE / INSTRUCTIONS	CERTIFICATE OF ANALYSIS	
	☐ Yes	☐ No

FORM
☐ Flower
☐ Edible
☐ Oil
☐ Tincture
☐ _____

METHOD
☐ Smoked
☐ Vaped
☐ Ingested
☐ Topical
☐ _____

CONTENT
____% CBD
____% THC
____% ____
____% ____
____% ____

VARIETY
☐ Indica
☐ Sativa
☐ Hybrid

Dose: _____ Smell / Taste: _____

Time to take effect: _____ Effect duration: _____

Reliefs
Pain:	① ② ③ ④ ⑤	Stress:	① ② ③ ④ ⑤
Nausea:	① ② ③ ④ ⑤	Anxiety:	① ② ③ ④ ⑤
Inflammation:	① ② ③ ④ ⑤	Insomnia:	① ② ③ ④ ⑤
Appetite:	① ② ③ ④ ⑤	Depression:	① ② ③ ④ ⑤

Other positive effects: _____

Adverse effects
Anxiety:	① ② ③ ④ ⑤	Dry Mouth:	① ② ③ ④ ⑤
Munchies:	① ② ③ ④ ⑤	Fatigue:	① ② ③ ④ ⑤

Other adverse effects: _____

Notes

My Rating: 🌿 🌿 🌿 🌿 🌿

Strain:_____ Distributor:_____

PRICE: _____

TOTAL ACQUIRED: _____

PURCHASE DATE: _____

DISTRIBUTOR #: _____

description / notes

DOSAGE / INSTRUCTIONS	CERTIFICATE OF ANALYSIS	
	☐ Yes	☐ No

FORM
☐ Flower
☐ Edible
☐ Oil
☐ Tincture
☐ _____

METHOD
☐ Smoked
☐ Vaped
☐ Ingested
☐ Topical
☐ _____

CONTENT
_____% CBD
_____% THC
_____% _____
_____% _____
_____% _____

VARIETY
☐ Indica
☐ Sativa
☐ Hybrid

Dose: _____ Smell / Taste: _____

Time to take effect: _____ Effect duration: _____

Reliefs

Pain:	① ② ③ ④ ⑤	Stress:	① ② ③ ④ ⑤
Nausea:	① ② ③ ④ ⑤	Anxiety:	① ② ③ ④ ⑤
Inflammation:	① ② ③ ④ ⑤	Insomnia:	① ② ③ ④ ⑤
Appetite:	① ② ③ ④ ⑤	Depression:	① ② ③ ④ ⑤

Other positive effects: _____

Adverse effects

Anxiety:	① ② ③ ④ ⑤	Dry Mouth:	① ② ③ ④ ⑤
Munchies:	① ② ③ ④ ⑤	Fatigue:	① ② ③ ④ ⑤

Other adverse effects: _____

Notes

My Rating: 🍁 🍁 🍁 🍁 🍁

DATE:	ENTRY:	70

Strain:_____ Distributor:_____

PRICE: _____
TOTAL ACQUIRED: _____
PURCHASE DATE: _____
DISTRIBUTOR #: _____

description / notes

DOSAGE / INSTRUCTIONS	CERTIFICATE OF ANALYSIS	
	☐ Yes	☐ No

FORM
☐ Flower
☐ Edible
☐ Oil
☐ Tincture
☐ _____

METHOD
☐ Smoked
☐ Vaped
☐ Ingested
☐ Topical
☐ _____

CONTENT
_____% CBD
_____% THC
_____% _____
_____% _____
_____% _____

VARIETY
☐ Indica
☐ Sativa
☐ Hybrid

Dose: _____ Smell / Taste: _____

Time to take effect: _____ Effect duration: _____

Reliefs
Pain:	① ② ③ ④ ⑤	Stress:	① ② ③ ④ ⑤
Nausea:	① ② ③ ④ ⑤	Anxiety:	① ② ③ ④ ⑤
Inflammation:	① ② ③ ④ ⑤	Insomnia:	① ② ③ ④ ⑤
Appetite:	① ② ③ ④ ⑤	Depression:	① ② ③ ④ ⑤

Other positive effects: _____

Adverse effects
Anxiety:	① ② ③ ④ ⑤	Dry Mouth:	① ② ③ ④ ⑤
Munchies:	① ② ③ ④ ⑤	Fatigue:	① ② ③ ④ ⑤

Other adverse effects: _____

Notes
_____
_____

My Rating: 🍁 🍁 🍁 🍁 🍁

DATE:		ENTRY:	71

Strain:_____ Distributor:_____

PRICE: _____

TOTAL ACQUIRED: _____

PURCHASE DATE: _____

DISTRIBUTOR #: _____

description / notes

DOSAGE / INSTRUCTIONS	CERTIFICATE OF ANALYSIS	
	☐ Yes	☐ No

FORM
☐ Flower
☐ Edible
☐ Oil
☐ Tincture
☐ _____

METHOD
☐ Smoked
☐ Vaped
☐ Ingested
☐ Topical
☐ _____

CONTENT
_____% CBD
_____% THC
_____% _____
_____% _____
_____% _____

VARIETY
☐ Indica
☐ Sativa
☐ Hybrid

Dose: _____   Smell / Taste: _____

Time to take effect: _____   Effect duration: _____

Reliefs

Pain:	①	②	③	④	⑤	Stress:	①	②	③	④	⑤
Nausea:	①	②	③	④	⑤	Anxiety:	①	②	③	④	⑤
Inflammation:	①	②	③	④	⑤	Insomnia:	①	②	③	④	⑤
Appetite:	①	②	③	④	⑤	Depression:	①	②	③	④	⑤

Other positive effects: _____

Adverse effects

Anxiety:	①	②	③	④	⑤	Dry Mouth:	①	②	③	④	⑤
Munchies:	①	②	③	④	⑤	Fatigue:	①	②	③	④	⑤

Other adverse effects: _____

Notes

My Rating: 🍁🍁🍁🍁🍁

Strain: _____ Distributor: _____

PRICE: _____	*description / notes*
TOTAL ACQUIRED: _____	
PURCHASE DATE: _____	
DISTRIBUTOR #: _____	

DOSAGE / INSTRUCTIONS	CERTIFICATE OF ANALYSIS	
	☐ Yes	☐ No

FORM
☐ Flower
☐ Edible
☐ Oil
☐ Tincture
☐ _____

METHOD
☐ Smoked
☐ Vaped
☐ Ingested
☐ Topical
☐ _____

CONTENT
_____% CBD
_____% THC
_____% _____
_____% _____
_____% _____

VARIETY
☐ Indica
☐ Sativa
☐ Hybrid

Dose: _____   Smell / Taste: _____

Time to take effect: _____   Effect duration: _____

Reliefs

Pain:	① ② ③ ④ ⑤	Stress:	① ② ③ ④ ⑤
Nausea:	① ② ③ ④ ⑤	Anxiety:	① ② ③ ④ ⑤
Inflammation:	① ② ③ ④ ⑤	Insomnia:	① ② ③ ④ ⑤
Appetite:	① ② ③ ④ ⑤	Depression:	① ② ③ ④ ⑤

Other positive effects: _____

Adverse effects

Anxiety:	① ② ③ ④ ⑤	Dry Mouth:	① ② ③ ④ ⑤
Munchies:	① ② ③ ④ ⑤	Fatigue:	① ② ③ ④ ⑤

Other adverse effects: _____

Notes

My Rating: 🍁 🍁 🍁 🍁 🍁

Strain:_____ Distributor:_____

PRICE: _____
TOTAL ACQUIRED: _____
PURCHASE DATE: _____
DISTRIBUTOR #: _____

description / notes

DOSAGE / INSTRUCTIONS	CERTIFICATE OF ANALYSIS	
	☐ Yes	☐ No

FORM
☐ Flower
☐ Edible
☐ Oil
☐ Tincture
☐ _____

METHOD
☐ Smoked
☐ Vaped
☐ Ingested
☐ Topical
☐ _____

CONTENT
_____% CBD
_____% THC
_____% _____
_____% _____
_____% _____

VARIETY
☐ Indica
☐ Sativa
☐ Hybrid

Dose: _____ Smell / Taste: _____

Time to take effect: _____ Effect duration: _____

Reliefs

Pain: ① ② ③ ④ ⑤   Stress: ① ② ③ ④ ⑤
Nausea: ① ② ③ ④ ⑤   Anxiety: ① ② ③ ④ ⑤
Inflammation: ① ② ③ ④ ⑤   Insomnia: ① ② ③ ④ ⑤
Appetite: ① ② ③ ④ ⑤   Depression: ① ② ③ ④ ⑤

Other positive effects: _____

Adverse effects

Anxiety: ① ② ③ ④ ⑤   Dry Mouth: ① ② ③ ④ ⑤
Munchies: ① ② ③ ④ ⑤   Fatigue: ① ② ③ ④ ⑤

Other adverse effects: _____

Notes

My Rating: 🍁 🍁 🍁 🍁 🍁

Strain:_____ Distributor:_____

PRICE: _____
TOTAL ACQUIRED: _____
PURCHASE DATE: _____
DISTRIBUTOR #: _____

description / notes

DOSAGE / INSTRUCTIONS	CERTIFICATE OF ANALYSIS	
	☐ Yes	☐ No

FORM
☐ Flower
☐ Edible
☐ Oil
☐ Tincture
☐ _____

METHOD
☐ Smoked
☐ Vaped
☐ Ingested
☐ Topical
☐ _____

CONTENT
_____% CBD
_____% THC
_____% _____
_____% _____
_____% _____

VARIETY
☐ Indica
☐ Sativa
☐ Hybrid

Dose: _____ Smell / Taste: _____

Time to take effect: _____ Effect duration: _____

Reliefs

Pain:	① ② ③ ④ ⑤	Stress:	① ② ③ ④ ⑤
Nausea:	① ② ③ ④ ⑤	Anxiety:	① ② ③ ④ ⑤
Inflammation:	① ② ③ ④ ⑤	Insomnia:	① ② ③ ④ ⑤
Appetite:	① ② ③ ④ ⑤	Depression:	① ② ③ ④ ⑤

Other positive effects: _____

Adverse effects

Anxiety:	① ② ③ ④ ⑤	Dry Mouth:	① ② ③ ④ ⑤
Munchies:	① ② ③ ④ ⑤	Fatigue:	① ② ③ ④ ⑤

Other adverse effects: _____

Notes

My Rating: 🍁 🍁 🍁 🍁 🍁

Strain:_____ Distributor:_____

PRICE: _____

TOTAL ACQUIRED: _____

PURCHASE DATE: _____

DISTRIBUTOR #: _____

description / notes

DOSAGE / INSTRUCTIONS	CERTIFICATE OF ANALYSIS	
	☐ Yes	☐ No

FORM
☐ Flower
☐ Edible
☐ Oil
☐ Tincture
☐ _____

METHOD
☐ Smoked
☐ Vaped
☐ Ingested
☐ Topical
☐ _____

CONTENT
_____% CBD
_____% THC
_____% _____
_____% _____
_____% _____

VARIETY
☐ Indica
☐ Sativa
☐ Hybrid

Dose: _____   Smell / Taste: _____

Time to take effect: _____   Effect duration: _____

Reliefs

Pain:	① ② ③ ④ ⑤					Stress:	① ② ③ ④ ⑤				
Nausea:	① ② ③ ④ ⑤					Anxiety:	① ② ③ ④ ⑤				
Inflammation:	① ② ③ ④ ⑤					Insomnia:	① ② ③ ④ ⑤				
Appetite:	① ② ③ ④ ⑤					Depression:	① ② ③ ④ ⑤				

Other positive effects: _____

Adverse effects

			Dry Mouth:	① ② ③ ④ ⑤
Anxiety:	① ② ③ ④ ⑤		Dry Mouth:	① ② ③ ④ ⑤
Munchies:	① ② ③ ④ ⑤		Fatigue:	① ② ③ ④ ⑤

Other adverse effects: _____

Notes

My Rating: 🍁 🍁 🍁 🍁 🍁

Strain:_____ Distributor:_____

PRICE: _____

TOTAL ACQUIRED: _____

PURCHASE DATE: _____

DISTRIBUTOR #: _____

description / notes

DOSAGE / INSTRUCTIONS	CERTIFICATE OF ANALYSIS	
	☐ Yes	☐ No

FORM
☐ Flower
☐ Edible
☐ Oil
☐ Tincture
☐ _____

METHOD
☐ Smoked
☐ Vaped
☐ Ingested
☐ Topical
☐ _____

CONTENT
_____% CBD
_____% THC
_____% _____
_____% _____
_____% _____

VARIETY
☐ Indica
☐ Sativa
☐ Hybrid

Dose: _____ Smell / Taste: _____

Time to take effect: _____ Effect duration: _____

Reliefs

Pain:	1	2	3	4	5	Stress:	1	2	3	4 5
Nausea:	1	2	3	4	5	Anxiety:	1	2	3	4 5
Inflammation:	1	2	3	4	5	Insomnia:	1	2	3	4 5
Appetite:	1	2	3	4	5	Depression:	1	2	3	4 5

Other positive effects: _____

Adverse effects

Anxiety:	1	2	3	4	5	Dry Mouth:	1	2	3	4 5
Munchies:	1	2	3	4	5	Fatigue:	1	2	3	4 5

Other adverse effects: _____

Notes

My Rating:

Strain:_____   Distributor:_____

PRICE: _____

TOTAL ACQUIRED: _____

PURCHASE DATE: _____

DISTRIBUTOR #: _____

description / notes

DOSAGE / INSTRUCTIONS	CERTIFICATE OF ANALYSIS
	☐ Yes ☐ No

FORM
☐ Flower
☐ Edible
☐ Oil
☐ Tincture
☐ _____

METHOD
☐ Smoked
☐ Vaped
☐ Ingested
☐ Topical
☐ _____

CONTENT
_____% CBD
_____% THC
_____% _____
_____% _____
_____% _____

VARIETY
☐ Indica
☐ Sativa
☐ Hybrid

Dose: _____   Smell / Taste: _____

Time to take effect: _____   Effect duration: _____

Reliefs

Pain: ① ② ③ ④ ⑤   Stress: ① ② ③ ④ ⑤

Nausea: ① ② ③ ④ ⑤   Anxiety: ① ② ③ ④ ⑤

Inflammation: ① ② ③ ④ ⑤   Insomnia: ① ② ③ ④ ⑤

Appetite: ① ② ③ ④ ⑤   Depression: ① ② ③ ④ ⑤

Other positive effects: _____

Adverse effects

Anxiety: ① ② ③ ④ ⑤   Dry Mouth: ① ② ③ ④ ⑤

Munchies: ① ② ③ ④ ⑤   Fatigue: ① ② ③ ④ ⑤

Other adverse effects: _____

Notes

My Rating: 🍁 🍁 🍁 🍁 🍁

DATE:		ENTRY:	78

Strain:_____ Distributor:_____

PRICE: _____

TOTAL ACQUIRED: _____

PURCHASE DATE: _____

DISTRIBUTOR #: _____

description / notes

DOSAGE / INSTRUCTIONS	CERTIFICATE OF ANALYSIS	
	☐ Yes	☐ No

FORM
☐ Flower
☐ Edible
☐ Oil
☐ Tincture
☐ _____

METHOD
☐ Smoked
☐ Vaped
☐ Ingested
☐ Topical
☐ _____

CONTENT
_____% CBD
_____% THC
_____% _____
_____% _____
_____% _____

VARIETY
☐ Indica
☐ Sativa
☐ Hybrid

Dose: _____   Smell / Taste: _____

Time to take effect: _____   Effect duration: _____

Reliefs

Pain: ① ② ③ ④ ⑤   Stress: ① ② ③ ④ ⑤

Nausea: ① ② ③ ④ ⑤   Anxiety: ① ② ③ ④ ⑤

Inflammation: ① ② ③ ④ ⑤   Insomnia: ① ② ③ ④ ⑤

Appetite: ① ② ③ ④ ⑤   Depression: ① ② ③ ④ ⑤

Other positive effects: _____

Adverse effects

Anxiety: ① ② ③ ④ ⑤   Dry Mouth: ① ② ③ ④ ⑤

Munchies: ① ② ③ ④ ⑤   Fatigue: ① ② ③ ④ ⑤

Other adverse effects: _____

Notes

My Rating: 🍁 🍁 🍁 🍁 🍁

Strain:_____ Distributor:_____

PRICE: _____
TOTAL ACQUIRED: _____
PURCHASE DATE: _____
DISTRIBUTOR #: _____

description / notes

DOSAGE / INSTRUCTIONS	CERTIFICATE OF ANALYSIS
	☐ Yes ☐ No

FORM
☐ Flower
☐ Edible
☐ Oil
☐ Tincture
☐ _____

METHOD
☐ Smoked
☐ Vaped
☐ Ingested
☐ Topical
☐ _____

CONTENT
_____% CBD
_____% THC
_____% _____
_____% _____
_____% _____

VARIETY
☐ Indica
☐ Sativa
☐ Hybrid

Dose: _____ Smell / Taste: _____

Time to take effect: _____ Effect duration: _____

Reliefs

Pain:	①	②	③	④	⑤	Stress:	①	②	③	④	⑤
Nausea:	①	②	③	④	⑤	Anxiety:	①	②	③	④	⑤
Inflammation:	①	②	③	④	⑤	Insomnia:	①	②	③	④	⑤
Appetite:	①	②	③	④	⑤	Depression:	①	②	③	④	⑤

Other positive effects: _____

Adverse effects

Anxiety:	①	②	③	④	⑤	Dry Mouth:	①	②	③	④	⑤
Munchies:	①	②	③	④	⑤	Fatigue:	①	②	③	④	⑤

Other adverse effects: _____

Notes

My Rating:

Strain: _____ Distributor: _____

PRICE: _____
TOTAL ACQUIRED: _____
PURCHASE DATE: _____
DISTRIBUTOR #: _____

description / notes

DOSAGE / INSTRUCTIONS	CERTIFICATE OF ANALYSIS	
	☐ Yes	☐ No

FORM
☐ Flower
☐ Edible
☐ Oil
☐ Tincture
☐ _____

METHOD
☐ Smoked
☐ Vaped
☐ Ingested
☐ Topical
☐ _____

CONTENT
____% CBD
____% THC
____% _____
____% _____
____% _____

VARIETY
☐ Indica
☐ Sativa
☐ Hybrid

Dose: _____ Smell / Taste: _____

Time to take effect: _____ Effect duration: _____

Reliefs

Pain:	① ② ③ ④ ⑤	Stress:	① ② ③ ④ ⑤
Nausea:	① ② ③ ④ ⑤	Anxiety:	① ② ③ ④ ⑤
Inflammation:	① ② ③ ④ ⑤	Insomnia:	① ② ③ ④ ⑤
Appetite:	① ② ③ ④ ⑤	Depression:	① ② ③ ④ ⑤

Other positive effects: _____

Adverse effects

Anxiety:	① ② ③ ④ ⑤	Dry Mouth:	① ② ③ ④ ⑤
Munchies:	① ② ③ ④ ⑤	Fatigue:	① ② ③ ④ ⑤

Other adverse effects: _____

Notes

My Rating: 🍁 🍁 🍁 🍁 🍁

Strain:_____ Distributor:_____

PRICE: _____

TOTAL ACQUIRED: _____

PURCHASE DATE: _____

DISTRIBUTOR #: _____

description / notes

DOSAGE / INSTRUCTIONS	CERTIFICATE OF ANALYSIS	
	☐ Yes	☐ No

FORM
☐ Flower
☐ Edible
☐ Oil
☐ Tincture
☐ _____

METHOD
☐ Smoked
☐ Vaped
☐ Ingested
☐ Topical
☐ _____

CONTENT
_____% CBD
_____% THC
_____% _____
_____% _____
_____% _____

VARIETY
☐ Indica
☐ Sativa
☐ Hybrid

Dose: _____ Smell / Taste: _____

Time to take effect: _____ Effect duration: _____

Reliefs

Pain: ① ② ③ ④ ⑤   Stress: ① ② ③ ④ ⑤

Nausea: ① ② ③ ④ ⑤   Anxiety: ① ② ③ ④ ⑤

Inflammation: ① ② ③ ④ ⑤   Insomnia: ① ② ③ ④ ⑤

Appetite: ① ② ③ ④ ⑤   Depression: ① ② ③ ④ ⑤

Other positive effects: _____

Adverse effects

Anxiety: ① ② ③ ④ ⑤   Dry Mouth: ① ② ③ ④ ⑤

Munchies: ① ② ③ ④ ⑤   Fatigue: ① ② ③ ④ ⑤

Other adverse effects: _____

Notes

My Rating: 🍁 🍁 🍁 🍁 🍁

Strain:_____ Distributor:_____

PRICE: _____
TOTAL ACQUIRED: _____
PURCHASE DATE: _____
DISTRIBUTOR #: _____

description / notes

DOSAGE / INSTRUCTIONS	CERTIFICATE OF ANALYSIS	
	☐ Yes	☐ No

FORM
☐ Flower
☐ Edible
☐ Oil
☐ Tincture
☐ _____

METHOD
☐ Smoked
☐ Vaped
☐ Ingested
☐ Topical
☐ _____

CONTENT
____% CBD
____% THC
____% ____
____% ____
____% ____

VARIETY
☐ Indica
☐ Sativa
☐ Hybrid

Dose: _____ Smell / Taste: _____

Time to take effect: _____ Effect duration: _____

Reliefs

Pain:	① ② ③ ④ ⑤	Stress:	① ② ③ ④ ⑤
Nausea:	① ② ③ ④ ⑤	Anxiety:	① ② ③ ④ ⑤
Inflammation:	① ② ③ ④ ⑤	Insomnia:	① ② ③ ④ ⑤
Appetite:	① ② ③ ④ ⑤	Depression:	① ② ③ ④ ⑤

Other positive effects: _____

Adverse effects

Anxiety:	① ② ③ ④ ⑤	Dry Mouth:	① ② ③ ④ ⑤
Munchies:	① ② ③ ④ ⑤	Fatigue:	① ② ③ ④ ⑤

Other adverse effects: _____

Notes

My Rating: ✿ ✿ ✿ ✿ ✿

DATE:	ENTRY:	83

Strain:_____ Distributor:_____

PRICE: _____
TOTAL ACQUIRED: _____
PURCHASE DATE: _____
DISTRIBUTOR #: _____

description / notes

DOSAGE / INSTRUCTIONS	CERTIFICATE OF ANALYSIS	
	☐ Yes	☐ No

FORM
☐ Flower
☐ Edible
☐ Oil
☐ Tincture
☐ _____

METHOD
☐ Smoked
☐ Vaped
☐ Ingested
☐ Topical
☐ _____

CONTENT
_____% CBD
_____% THC
_____% _____
_____% _____
_____% _____

VARIETY
☐ Indica
☐ Sativa
☐ Hybrid

Dose: _____ Smell / Taste: _____

Time to take effect: _____ Effect duration: _____

Reliefs

Pain:	① ② ③ ④ ⑤	Stress:	① ② ③ ④ ⑤
Nausea:	① ② ③ ④ ⑤	Anxiety:	① ② ③ ④ ⑤
Inflammation:	① ② ③ ④ ⑤	Insomnia:	① ② ③ ④ ⑤
Appetite:	① ② ③ ④ ⑤	Depression:	① ② ③ ④ ⑤

Other positive effects: _____

Adverse effects

Anxiety:	① ② ③ ④ ⑤	Dry Mouth:	① ② ③ ④ ⑤
Munchies:	① ② ③ ④ ⑤	Fatigue:	① ② ③ ④ ⑤

Other adverse effects: _____

Notes

My Rating: 🍁 🍁 🍁 🍁 🍁

Strain:_____ Distributor:_____

PRICE: _____

TOTAL ACQUIRED: _____

PURCHASE DATE: _____

DISTRIBUTOR #: _____

description / notes

DOSAGE / INSTRUCTIONS	CERTIFICATE OF ANALYSIS	
	☐ Yes	☐ No

FORM
☐ Flower
☐ Edible
☐ Oil
☐ Tincture
☐ _____

METHOD
☐ Smoked
☐ Vaped
☐ Ingested
☐ Topical
☐ _____

CONTENT
_____% CBD
_____% THC
_____% _____
_____% _____
_____% _____

VARIETY
☐ Indica
☐ Sativa
☐ Hybrid

Dose: _____   Smell / Taste: _____

Time to take effect: _____   Effect duration: _____

Reliefs

Pain:	①	②	③	④	⑤	Stress:	①	②	③	④	⑤
Nausea:	①	②	③	④	⑤	Anxiety:	①	②	③	④	⑤
Inflammation:	①	②	③	④	⑤	Insomnia:	①	②	③	④	⑤
Appetite:	①	②	③	④	⑤	Depression:	①	②	③	④	⑤

Other positive effects: _____

Adverse effects

Anxiety:	①	②	③	④	⑤	Dry Mouth:	①	②	③	④	⑤
Munchies:	①	②	③	④	⑤	Fatigue:	①	②	③	④	⑤

Other adverse effects: _____

Notes

_____

My Rating: 🍁 🍁 🍁 🍁 🍁

DATE:	ENTRY:	85

Strain:_____ Distributor:_____

PRICE: _____
TOTAL ACQUIRED: _____
PURCHASE DATE: _____
DISTRIBUTOR #: _____

description / notes

DOSAGE / INSTRUCTIONS	CERTIFICATE OF ANALYSIS	
	☐ Yes	☐ No

FORM
☐ Flower
☐ Edible
☐ Oil
☐ Tincture
☐ _____

METHOD
☐ Smoked
☐ Vaped
☐ Ingested
☐ Topical
☐ _____

CONTENT
_____% CBD
_____% THC
_____% _____
_____% _____
_____% _____

VARIETY
☐ Indica
☐ Sativa
☐ Hybrid

Dose: _____ Smell / Taste: _____

Time to take effect: _____ Effect duration: _____

Reliefs

Pain:	①	②	③	④	⑤	Stress:	①	②	③	④	⑤
Nausea:	①	②	③	④	⑤	Anxiety:	①	②	③	④	⑤
Inflammation:	①	②	③	④	⑤	Insomnia:	①	②	③	④	⑤
Appetite:	①	②	③	④	⑤	Depression:	①	②	③	④	⑤

Other positive effects: _____

Adverse effects

Anxiety:	①	②	③	④	⑤	Dry Mouth:	①	②	③	④	⑤
Munchies:	①	②	③	④	⑤	Fatigue:	①	②	③	④	⑤

Other adverse effects: _____

Notes

My Rating: 🍁 🍁 🍁 🍁 🍁

Strain:_____ Distributor:_____

PRICE: _____
TOTAL ACQUIRED: _____
PURCHASE DATE: _____
DISTRIBUTOR #: _____

description / notes

DOSAGE / INSTRUCTIONS	CERTIFICATE OF ANALYSIS	
	☐ Yes	☐ No

FORM
☐ Flower
☐ Edible
☐ Oil
☐ Tincture
☐ _____

METHOD
☐ Smoked
☐ Vaped
☐ Ingested
☐ Topical
☐ _____

CONTENT
_____% CBD
_____% THC
_____% _____
_____% _____
_____% _____

VARIETY
☐ Indica
☐ Sativa
☐ Hybrid

Dose: _____   Smell / Taste: _____

Time to take effect: _____   Effect duration: _____

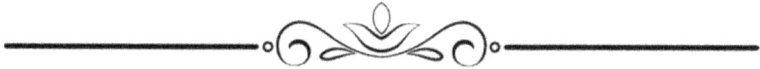

Reliefs

Pain: ① ② ③ ④ ⑤   Stress: ① ② ③ ④ ⑤
Nausea: ① ② ③ ④ ⑤   Anxiety: ① ② ③ ④ ⑤
Inflammation: ① ② ③ ④ ⑤   Insomnia: ① ② ③ ④ ⑤
Appetite: ① ② ③ ④ ⑤   Depression: ① ② ③ ④ ⑤

Other positive effects: _____

Adverse effects

Anxiety: ① ② ③ ④ ⑤   Dry Mouth: ① ② ③ ④ ⑤
Munchies: ① ② ③ ④ ⑤   Fatigue: ① ② ③ ④ ⑤

Other adverse effects: _____

Notes

My Rating: 🍁 🍁 🍁 🍁 🍁

DATE:	ENTRY:	87

Strain:_____ Distributor:_____

PRICE: _____

TOTAL ACQUIRED: _____

PURCHASE DATE: _____

DISTRIBUTOR #: _____

description / notes

DOSAGE / INSTRUCTIONS	CERTIFICATE OF ANALYSIS	
	☐ Yes	☐ No

FORM
☐ Flower
☐ Edible
☐ Oil
☐ Tincture
☐ _____

METHOD
☐ Smoked
☐ Vaped
☐ Ingested
☐ Topical
☐ _____

CONTENT
_____% CBD
_____% THC
_____% _____
_____% _____
_____% _____

VARIETY
☐ Indica
☐ Sativa
☐ Hybrid

Dose: _____ Smell / Taste: _____

Time to take effect: _____ Effect duration: _____

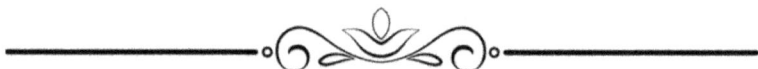

Reliefs

Pain:	①②③④⑤	Stress:	①②③④⑤
Nausea:	①②③④⑤	Anxiety:	①②③④⑤
Inflammation:	①②③④⑤	Insomnia:	①②③④⑤
Appetite:	①②③④⑤	Depression:	①②③④⑤

Other positive effects: _____

Adverse effects

Anxiety:	①②③④⑤	Dry Mouth:	①②③④⑤
Munchies:	①②③④⑤	Fatigue:	①②③④⑤

Other adverse effects: _____

Notes

My Rating: 🍁🍁🍁🍁🍁

DATE:		ENTRY:	88

Strain:_____ Distributor:_____

PRICE: _____
TOTAL ACQUIRED: _____
PURCHASE DATE: _____
DISTRIBUTOR #: _____

description / notes

DOSAGE / INSTRUCTIONS	CERTIFICATE OF ANALYSIS	
	☐ Yes	☐ No

FORM
☐ Flower
☐ Edible
☐ Oil
☐ Tincture
☐ _____

METHOD
☐ Smoked
☐ Vaped
☐ Ingested
☐ Topical
☐ _____

CONTENT
_____% CBD
_____% THC
_____% _____
_____% _____
_____% _____

VARIETY
☐ Indica
☐ Sativa
☐ Hybrid

Dose: _____   Smell / Taste: _____

Time to take effect: _____   Effect duration: _____

Reliefs
Pain: ① ② ③ ④ ⑤   Stress: ① ② ③ ④ ⑤
Nausea: ① ② ③ ④ ⑤   Anxiety: ① ② ③ ④ ⑤
Inflammation: ① ② ③ ④ ⑤   Insomnia: ① ② ③ ④ ⑤
Appetite: ① ② ③ ④ ⑤   Depression: ① ② ③ ④ ⑤

Other positive effects: _____

Adverse effects
Anxiety: ① ② ③ ④ ⑤   Dry Mouth: ① ② ③ ④ ⑤
Munchies: ① ② ③ ④ ⑤   Fatigue: ① ② ③ ④ ⑤

Other adverse effects: _____

Notes
_____

My Rating: ✿ ✿ ✿ ✿ ✿

Strain:_____ Distributor:_____

PRICE: _____
TOTAL ACQUIRED: _____
PURCHASE DATE: _____
DISTRIBUTOR #: _____

description / notes

DOSAGE / INSTRUCTIONS	CERTIFICATE OF ANALYSIS	
	☐ Yes	☐ No

FORM
☐ Flower
☐ Edible
☐ Oil
☐ Tincture
☐ _____

METHOD
☐ Smoked
☐ Vaped
☐ Ingested
☐ Topical
☐ _____

CONTENT
_____% CBD
_____% THC
_____% _____
_____% _____
_____% _____

VARIETY
☐ Indica
☐ Sativa
☐ Hybrid

Dose: _____   Smell / Taste: _____

Time to take effect: _____   Effect duration: _____

Reliefs

Pain:	① ② ③ ④ ⑤	Stress:	① ② ③ ④ ⑤
Nausea:	① ② ③ ④ ⑤	Anxiety:	① ② ③ ④ ⑤
Inflammation:	① ② ③ ④ ⑤	Insomnia:	① ② ③ ④ ⑤
Appetite:	① ② ③ ④ ⑤	Depression:	① ② ③ ④ ⑤

Other positive effects: _____

Adverse effects

Anxiety:	① ② ③ ④ ⑤	Dry Mouth:	① ② ③ ④ ⑤
Munchies:	① ② ③ ④ ⑤	Fatigue:	① ② ③ ④ ⑤

Other adverse effects: _____

Notes

My Rating: ✺ ✺ ✺ ✺ ✺

Strain:_____ Distributor:_____

PRICE: _____
TOTAL ACQUIRED: _____
PURCHASE DATE: _____
DISTRIBUTOR #: _____

description / notes

DOSAGE / INSTRUCTIONS	CERTIFICATE OF ANALYSIS	
	☐ Yes	☐ No

FORM
☐ Flower
☐ Edible
☐ Oil
☐ Tincture
☐ _____

METHOD
☐ Smoked
☐ Vaped
☐ Ingested
☐ Topical
☐ _____

CONTENT
_____% CBD
_____% THC
_____% _____
_____% _____
_____% _____

VARIETY
☐ Indica
☐ Sativa
☐ Hybrid

Dose: _____ Smell / Taste: _____

Time to take effect: _____ Effect duration: _____

Reliefs

Pain:	①	②	③	④	⑤	Stress:	①	②	③	④	⑤
Nausea:	①	②	③	④	⑤	Anxiety:	①	②	③	④	⑤
Inflammation:	①	②	③	④	⑤	Insomnia:	①	②	③	④	⑤
Appetite:	①	②	③	④	⑤	Depression:	①	②	③	④	⑤

Other positive effects: _____

Adverse effects

Anxiety:	①	②	③	④	⑤	Dry Mouth:	①	②	③	④	⑤
Munchies:	①	②	③	④	⑤	Fatigue:	①	②	③	④	⑤

Other adverse effects: _____

Notes

_____
_____

My Rating: 🍁 🍁 🍁 🍁 🍁

Strain:_____ Distributor:_____

PRICE: _____

TOTAL ACQUIRED: _____

PURCHASE DATE: _____

DISTRIBUTOR #: _____

description / notes

DOSAGE / INSTRUCTIONS	CERTIFICATE OF ANALYSIS	
	☐ Yes	☐ No

FORM
☐ Flower
☐ Edible
☐ Oil
☐ Tincture
☐ _____

METHOD
☐ Smoked
☐ Vaped
☐ Ingested
☐ Topical
☐ _____

CONTENT
_____% CBD
_____% THC
_____% _____
_____% _____
_____% _____

VARIETY
☐ Indica
☐ Sativa
☐ Hybrid

Dose: _____ Smell / Taste: _____

Time to take effect: _____ Effect duration: _____

Reliefs

Pain:	①	②	③	④	⑤	Stress:	①	②	③	④	⑤
Nausea:	①	②	③	④	⑤	Anxiety:	①	②	③	④	⑤
Inflammation:	①	②	③	④	⑤	Insomnia:	①	②	③	④	⑤
Appetite:	①	②	③	④	⑤	Depression:	①	②	③	④	⑤

Other positive effects: _____

Adverse effects

Anxiety:	①	②	③	④	⑤	Dry Mouth:	①	②	③	④	⑤
Munchies:	①	②	③	④	⑤	Fatigue:	①	②	③	④	⑤

Other adverse effects: _____

Notes

My Rating: 🍁 🍁 🍁 🍁 🍁

Strain:_____ Distributor:_____

PRICE: _____
TOTAL ACQUIRED: _____
PURCHASE DATE: _____
DISTRIBUTOR #: _____

description / notes

DOSAGE / INSTRUCTIONS	CERTIFICATE OF ANALYSIS	
	☐ Yes	☐ No

FORM
☐ Flower
☐ Edible
☐ Oil
☐ Tincture
☐ _____

METHOD
☐ Smoked
☐ Vaped
☐ Ingested
☐ Topical
☐ _____

CONTENT
_____% CBD
_____% THC
_____% _____
_____% _____
_____% _____

VARIETY
☐ Indica
☐ Sativa
☐ Hybrid

Dose: _____ Smell / Taste: _____

Time to take effect: _____ Effect duration: _____

Reliefs
Pain: ① ② ③ ④ ⑤   Stress: ① ② ③ ④ ⑤
Nausea: ① ② ③ ④ ⑤   Anxiety: ① ② ③ ④ ⑤
Inflammation: ① ② ③ ④ ⑤   Depression: ① ② ③ ④ ⑤
Appetite: ① ② ③ ④ ⑤   Insomnia: ① ② ③ ④ ⑤

Other positive effects: _____

Adverse effects
Anxiety: ① ② ③ ④ ⑤   Dry Mouth: ① ② ③ ④ ⑤
Munchies: ① ② ③ ④ ⑤   Fatigue: ① ② ③ ④ ⑤

Other adverse effects: _____

Notes

My Rating: 🍁 🍁 🍁 🍁 🍁

DATE:	ENTRY:	93

Strain:_____ Distributor:_____

PRICE: _____
TOTAL ACQUIRED: _____
PURCHASE DATE: _____
DISTRIBUTOR #: _____

description / notes

DOSAGE / INSTRUCTIONS	CERTIFICATE OF ANALYSIS	
	☐ Yes	☐ No

FORM
☐ Flower
☐ Edible
☐ Oil
☐ Tincture
☐ _____

METHOD
☐ Smoked
☐ Vaped
☐ Ingested
☐ Topical
☐ _____

CONTENT
_____% CBD
_____% THC
_____% _____
_____% _____
_____% _____

VARIETY
☐ Indica
☐ Sativa
☐ Hybrid

Dose: _____ Smell / Taste: _____

Time to take effect: _____ Effect duration: _____

Reliefs

Pain:	①	②	③	④	⑤	Stress:	①	②	③	④	⑤
Nausea:	①	②	③	④	⑤	Anxiety:	①	②	③	④	⑤
Inflammation:	①	②	③	④	⑤	Insomnia:	①	②	③	④	⑤
Appetite:	①	②	③	④	⑤	Depression:	①	②	③	④	⑤

Other positive effects: _____

Adverse effects

Anxiety:	①	②	③	④	⑤	Dry Mouth:	①	②	③	④	⑤
Munchies:	①	②	③	④	⑤	Fatigue:	①	②	③	④	⑤

Other adverse effects: _____

Notes

My Rating:

DATE:	ENTRY:	94

Strain:_____ Distributor:_____

PRICE: _____
TOTAL ACQUIRED: _____
PURCHASE DATE: _____
DISTRIBUTOR #: _____

description / notes

DOSAGE / INSTRUCTIONS	CERTIFICATE OF ANALYSIS	
	☐ Yes	☐ No

FORM
☐ Flower
☐ Edible
☐ Oil
☐ Tincture
☐ _____

METHOD
☐ Smoked
☐ Vaped
☐ Ingested
☐ Topical
☐ _____

CONTENT
_____% CBD
_____% THC
_____% _____
_____% _____
_____% _____

VARIETY
☐ Indica
☐ Sativa
☐ Hybrid

Dose: _____ Smell / Taste: _____

Time to take effect: _____ Effect duration: _____

Reliefs

Pain: ① ② ③ ④ ⑤   Stress: ① ② ③ ④ ⑤
Nausea: ① ② ③ ④ ⑤   Anxiety: ① ② ③ ④ ⑤
Inflammation: ① ② ③ ④ ⑤   Insomnia: ① ② ③ ④ ⑤
Appetite: ① ② ③ ④ ⑤   Depression: ① ② ③ ④ ⑤

Other positive effects: _____

Adverse effects

Anxiety: ① ② ③ ④ ⑤   Dry Mouth: ① ② ③ ④ ⑤
Munchies: ① ② ③ ④ ⑤   Fatigue: ① ② ③ ④ ⑤

Other adverse effects: _____

Notes

My Rating: 🍁🍁🍁🍁🍁

Strain:_____ Distributor:_____

PRICE: _____
TOTAL ACQUIRED: _____
PURCHASE DATE: _____
DISTRIBUTOR #: _____

description / notes

DOSAGE / INSTRUCTIONS	CERTIFICATE OF ANALYSIS
	☐ Yes ☐ No

FORM	METHOD	CONTENT	VARIETY
☐ Flower	☐ Smoked	_____% CBD	☐ Indica
☐ Edible	☐ Vaped	_____% THC	☐ Sativa
☐ Oil	☐ Ingested	_____% _____	☐ Hybrid
☐ Tincture	☐ Topical	_____% _____	
☐ _____	☐ _____	_____% _____	

Dose: _____ Smell / Taste: _____

Time to take effect: _____ Effect duration: _____

Reliefs

Pain: ① ② ③ ④ ⑤   Stress: ① ② ③ ④ ⑤

Nausea: ① ② ③ ④ ⑤   Anxiety: ① ② ③ ④ ⑤

Inflammation: ① ② ③ ④ ⑤   Insomnia: ① ② ③ ④ ⑤

Appetite: ① ② ③ ④ ⑤   Depression: ① ② ③ ④ ⑤

Other positive effects: _____

Adverse effects

Anxiety: ① ② ③ ④ ⑤   Dry Mouth: ① ② ③ ④ ⑤

Munchies: ① ② ③ ④ ⑤   Fatigue: ① ② ③ ④ ⑤

Other adverse effects: _____

Notes

My Rating: 🍁 🍁 🍁 🍁 🍁

DATE:		ENTRY:	96

Strain:_____ Distributor:_____

PRICE: _____
TOTAL ACQUIRED: _____
PURCHASE DATE: _____
DISTRIBUTOR #: _____

description / notes

DOSAGE / INSTRUCTIONS	CERTIFICATE OF ANALYSIS	
	☐ Yes	☐ No

FORM
☐ Flower
☐ Edible
☐ Oil
☐ Tincture
☐ _____

METHOD
☐ Smoked
☐ Vaped
☐ Ingested
☐ Topical
☐ _____

CONTENT
____% CBD
____% THC
____% ____
____% ____
____% ____

VARIETY
☐ Indica
☐ Sativa
☐ Hybrid

Dose: _____   Smell / Taste: _____

Time to take effect: _____   Effect duration: _____

Reliefs

Pain:	① ② ③ ④ ⑤					Stress:	① ② ③ ④ ⑤			
Nausea:	① ② ③ ④ ⑤					Anxiety:	① ② ③ ④ ⑤			
Inflammation:	① ② ③ ④ ⑤					Insomnia:	① ② ③ ④ ⑤			
Appetite:	① ② ③ ④ ⑤					Depression:	① ② ③ ④ ⑤			

Other positive effects: _____

Adverse effects

Anxiety:	① ② ③ ④ ⑤					Dry Mouth:	① ② ③ ④ ⑤			
Munchies:	① ② ③ ④ ⑤					Fatigue:	① ② ③ ④ ⑤			

Other adverse effects: _____

Notes
_____

My Rating: ✿ ✿ ✿ ✿ ✿

DATE:		ENTRY:	97

Strain:_____ Distributor:_____

PRICE: _____

TOTAL ACQUIRED: _____

PURCHASE DATE: _____

DISTRIBUTOR #: _____

description / notes

DOSAGE / INSTRUCTIONS	CERTIFICATE OF ANALYSIS	
	☐ Yes	☐ No

FORM
☐ Flower
☐ Edible
☐ Oil
☐ Tincture
☐ _____

METHOD
☐ Smoked
☐ Vaped
☐ Ingested
☐ Topical
☐ _____

CONTENT
_____% CBD
_____% THC
_____% _____
_____% _____
_____% _____

VARIETY
☐ Indica
☐ Sativa
☐ Hybrid

Dose: _____ Smell / Taste: _____

Time to take effect: _____ Effect duration: _____

Reliefs

Pain:	① ② ③ ④ ⑤	Stress:	① ② ③ ④ ⑤
Nausea:	① ② ③ ④ ⑤	Anxiety:	① ② ③ ④ ⑤
Inflammation:	① ② ③ ④ ⑤	Insomnia:	① ② ③ ④ ⑤
Appetite:	① ② ③ ④ ⑤	Depression:	① ② ③ ④ ⑤

Other positive effects: _____

Adverse effects

Anxiety:	① ② ③ ④ ⑤	Dry Mouth:	① ② ③ ④ ⑤
Munchies:	① ② ③ ④ ⑤	Fatigue:	① ② ③ ④ ⑤

Other adverse effects: _____

Notes

My Rating: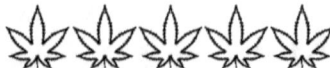

DATE:	ENTRY:	98

Strain:_____ Distributor:_____

PRICE: _____	*description / notes*
TOTAL ACQUIRED: _____	
PURCHASE DATE: _____	
DISTRIBUTOR #: _____	

DOSAGE / INSTRUCTIONS	CERTIFICATE OF ANALYSIS	
	☐ Yes	☐ No

FORM	METHOD	CONTENT	VARIETY
☐ Flower	☐ Smoked	_____% CBD	☐ Indica
☐ Edible	☐ Vaped	_____% THC	☐ Sativa
☐ Oil	☐ Ingested	_____% _____	☐ Hybrid
☐ Tincture	☐ Topical	_____% _____	
☐ _____	☐ _____	_____% _____	

Dose: _____   Smell / Taste: _____

Time to take effect: _____   Effect duration: _____

Reliefs

Pain:	1 2 3 4 5	Stress:	1 2 3 4 5
Nausea:	1 2 3 4 5	Anxiety:	1 2 3 4 5
Inflammation:	1 2 3 4 5	Insomnia:	1 2 3 4 5
Appetite:	1 2 3 4 5	Depression:	1 2 3 4 5

Other positive effects: _____

Adverse effects

Anxiety:	1 2 3 4 5	Dry Mouth:	1 2 3 4 5
Munchies:	1 2 3 4 5	Fatigue:	1 2 3 4 5

Other adverse effects: _____

Notes

My Rating: 🍁 🍁 🍁 🍁 🍁

| DATE: | | ENTRY: | 99 |

Strain:_____ Distributor:_____

PRICE: _____
TOTAL ACQUIRED: _____
PURCHASE DATE: _____
DISTRIBUTOR #: _____

description / notes

DOSAGE / INSTRUCTIONS	CERTIFICATE OF ANALYSIS	
	☐ Yes	☐ No

FORM	METHOD	CONTENT	VARIETY
☐ Flower	☐ Smoked	_____% CBD	☐ Indica
☐ Edible	☐ Vaped	_____% THC	☐ Sativa
☐ Oil	☐ Ingested	_____% _____	☐ Hybrid
☐ Tincture	☐ Topical	_____% _____	
☐ _____	☐ _____	_____% _____	

Dose: _____ Smell / Taste: _____

Time to take effect: _____ Effect duration: _____

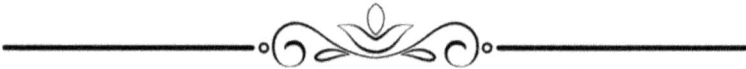

Reliefs

Pain: ① ② ③ ④ ⑤   Stress: ① ② ③ ④ ⑤
Nausea: ① ② ③ ④ ⑤   Anxiety: ① ② ③ ④ ⑤
Inflammation: ① ② ③ ④ ⑤   Insomnia: ① ② ③ ④ ⑤
Appetite: ① ② ③ ④ ⑤   Depression: ① ② ③ ④ ⑤

Other positive effects: _____

Adverse effects

Anxiety: ① ② ③ ④ ⑤   Dry Mouth: ① ② ③ ④ ⑤
Munchies: ① ② ③ ④ ⑤   Fatigue: ① ② ③ ④ ⑤

Other adverse effects: _____

Notes

My Rating: 🍁 🍁 🍁 🍁 🍁

Strain:_____ Distributor:_____

PRICE: _____

TOTAL ACQUIRED: _____

PURCHASE DATE: _____

DISTRIBUTOR #: _____

description / notes

DOSAGE / INSTRUCTIONS	CERTIFICATE OF ANALYSIS	
	☐ Yes	☐ No

FORM
☐ Flower
☐ Edible
☐ Oil
☐ Tincture
☐ _____

METHOD
☐ Smoked
☐ Vaped
☐ Ingested
☐ Topical
☐ _____

CONTENT
_____% CBD
_____% THC
_____% _____
_____% _____
_____% _____

VARIETY
☐ Indica
☐ Sativa
☐ Hybrid

Dose: _____ Smell / Taste: _____

Time to take effect: _____ Effect duration: _____

Reliefs

Pain: ① ② ③ ④ ⑤   Stress: ① ② ③ ④ ⑤

Nausea: ① ② ③ ④ ⑤   Anxiety: ① ② ③ ④ ⑤

Inflammation: ① ② ③ ④ ⑤   Insomnia: ① ② ③ ④ ⑤

Appetite: ① ② ③ ④ ⑤   Depression: ① ② ③ ④ ⑤

Other positive effects: _____

Adverse effects

Anxiety: ① ② ③ ④ ⑤   Dry Mouth: ① ② ③ ④ ⑤

Munchies: ① ② ③ ④ ⑤   Fatigue: ① ② ③ ④ ⑤

Other adverse effects: _____

Notes

My Rating: 🌿 🌿 🌿 🌿 🌿

Strain:_____ Distributor:_____

PRICE: _____

TOTAL ACQUIRED: _____

PURCHASE DATE: _____

DISTRIBUTOR #: _____

description / notes

DOSAGE / INSTRUCTIONS	CERTIFICATE OF ANALYSIS
	☐ Yes ☐ No

FORM
☐ Flower
☐ Edible
☐ Oil
☐ Tincture
☐ _____

METHOD
☐ Smoked
☐ Vaped
☐ Ingested
☐ Topical
☐ _____

CONTENT
_____% CBD
_____% THC
_____% _____
_____% _____
_____% _____

VARIETY
☐ Indica
☐ Sativa
☐ Hybrid

Dose: _____ Smell / Taste: _____

Time to take effect: _____ Effect duration: _____

Reliefs

Pain:	① ② ③ ④ ⑤	Stress:	① ② ③ ④ ⑤
Nausea:	① ② ③ ④ ⑤	Anxiety:	① ② ③ ④ ⑤
Inflammation:	① ② ③ ④ ⑤	Insomnia:	① ② ③ ④ ⑤
Appetite:	① ② ③ ④ ⑤	Depression:	① ② ③ ④ ⑤

Other positive effects: _____

Adverse effects

Anxiety:	① ② ③ ④ ⑤	Dry Mouth:	① ② ③ ④ ⑤
Munchies:	① ② ③ ④ ⑤	Fatigue:	① ② ③ ④ ⑤

Other adverse effects: _____

Notes

My Rating: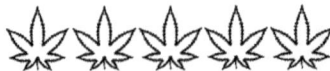

Strain:_____ Distributor:_____

PRICE: _____

TOTAL ACQUIRED: _____

PURCHASE DATE: _____

DISTRIBUTOR #: _____

description / notes

DOSAGE / INSTRUCTIONS	CERTIFICATE OF ANALYSIS	
	☐ Yes	☐ No

FORM
☐ Flower
☐ Edible
☐ Oil
☐ Tincture
☐ _____

METHOD
☐ Smoked
☐ Vaped
☐ Ingested
☐ Topical
☐ _____

CONTENT
_____% CBD
_____% THC
_____% _____
_____% _____
_____% _____

VARIETY
☐ Indica
☐ Sativa
☐ Hybrid

Dose: _____   Smell / Taste: _____

Time to take effect: _____   Effect duration: _____

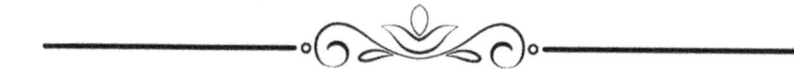

Reliefs

Pain:	①	②	③	④	⑤	Stress:	①	②	③	④	⑤
Nausea:	①	②	③	④	⑤	Anxiety:	①	②	③	④	⑤
Inflammation:	①	②	③	④	⑤	Insomnia:	①	②	③	④	⑤
Appetite:	①	②	③	④	⑤	Depression:	①	②	③	④	⑤

Other positive effects: _____

Adverse effects

Anxiety:	①	②	③	④	⑤	Dry Mouth:	①	②	③	④	⑤
Munchies:	①	②	③	④	⑤	Fatigue:	①	②	③	④	⑤

Other adverse effects: _____

Notes

My Rating: 🌿🌿🌿🌿🌿

Strain:_____ Distributor:_____

PRICE: _____

TOTAL ACQUIRED: _____

PURCHASE DATE: _____

DISTRIBUTOR #: _____

description / notes

DOSAGE / INSTRUCTIONS	CERTIFICATE OF ANALYSIS	
	☐ Yes	☐ No

FORM	METHOD	CONTENT	VARIETY
☐ Flower	☐ Smoked	_____% CBD	☐ Indica
☐ Edible	☐ Vaped	_____% THC	☐ Sativa
☐ Oil	☐ Ingested	_____% _____	☐ Hybrid
☐ Tincture	☐ Topical	_____% _____	
☐ _____	☐ _____	_____% _____	

Dose: _____ Smell / Taste: _____

Time to take effect: _____ Effect duration: _____

Reliefs

Pain:	① ② ③ ④ ⑤	Stress:	① ② ③ ④ ⑤
Nausea:	① ② ③ ④ ⑤	Anxiety:	① ② ③ ④ ⑤
Inflammation:	① ② ③ ④ ⑤	Insomnia:	① ② ③ ④ ⑤
Appetite:	① ② ③ ④ ⑤	Depression:	① ② ③ ④ ⑤

Other positive effects: _____

Adverse effects

Anxiety:	① ② ③ ④ ⑤	Dry Mouth:	① ② ③ ④ ⑤
Munchies:	① ② ③ ④ ⑤	Fatigue:	① ② ③ ④ ⑤

Other adverse effects: _____

Notes

My Rating:

Strain:_____ Distributor:_____

PRICE: _____
TOTAL ACQUIRED: _____
PURCHASE DATE: _____
DISTRIBUTOR #: _____

description / notes

DOSAGE / INSTRUCTIONS	CERTIFICATE OF ANALYSIS	
	☐ Yes	☐ No

FORM
☐ Flower
☐ Edible
☐ Oil
☐ Tincture
☐ _____

METHOD
☐ Smoked
☐ Vaped
☐ Ingested
☐ Topical
☐ _____

CONTENT
____% CBD
____% THC
____% ____
____% ____
____% ____

VARIETY
☐ Indica
☐ Sativa
☐ Hybrid

Dose: _____ Smell / Taste: _____

Time to take effect: _____ Effect duration: _____

Reliefs

Pain:	① ② ③ ④ ⑤	Stress:	① ② ③ ④ ⑤
Nausea:	① ② ③ ④ ⑤	Anxiety:	① ② ③ ④ ⑤
Inflammation:	① ② ③ ④ ⑤	Insomnia:	① ② ③ ④ ⑤
Appetite:	① ② ③ ④ ⑤	Depression:	① ② ③ ④ ⑤

Other positive effects: _____

Adverse effects

Anxiety:	① ② ③ ④ ⑤	Dry Mouth:	① ② ③ ④ ⑤
Munchies:	① ② ③ ④ ⑤	Fatigue:	① ② ③ ④ ⑤

Other adverse effects: _____

Notes

My Rating: 🍁🍁🍁🍁🍁

DATE:		ENTRY:	105

Strain:_____ Distributor:_____

PRICE: _____
TOTAL ACQUIRED: _____
PURCHASE DATE: _____
DISTRIBUTOR #: _____

description / notes

DOSAGE / INSTRUCTIONS	CERTIFICATE OF ANALYSIS	
	☐ Yes	☐ No

FORM	METHOD	CONTENT	VARIETY
☐ Flower	☐ Smoked	____% CBD	☐ Indica
☐ Edible	☐ Vaped	____% THC	☐ Sativa
☐ Oil	☐ Ingested	____% ____	☐ Hybrid
☐ Tincture	☐ Topical	____% ____	
☐ _____	☐ _____	____% ____	

Dose: _____ Smell / Taste: _____

Time to take effect: _____ Effect duration: _____

Reliefs

Pain:	① ② ③ ④ ⑤	Stress:	① ② ③ ④ ⑤
Nausea:	① ② ③ ④ ⑤	Anxiety:	① ② ③ ④ ⑤
Inflammation:	① ② ③ ④ ⑤	Insomnia:	① ② ③ ④ ⑤
Appetite:	① ② ③ ④ ⑤	Depression:	① ② ③ ④ ⑤

Other positive effects: _____

Adverse effects

Anxiety:	① ② ③ ④ ⑤	Dry Mouth:	① ② ③ ④ ⑤
Munchies:	① ② ③ ④ ⑤	Fatigue:	① ② ③ ④ ⑤

Other adverse effects: _____

Notes

My Rating: 🍁 🍁 🍁 🍁 🍁

DATE:		ENTRY:	106

Strain:_____ Distributor:_____

PRICE: _____

TOTAL ACQUIRED: _____

PURCHASE DATE: _____

DISTRIBUTOR #: _____

description / notes

DOSAGE / INSTRUCTIONS	CERTIFICATE OF ANALYSIS	
	☐ Yes	☐ No

FORM
☐ Flower
☐ Edible
☐ Oil
☐ Tincture
☐ _____

METHOD
☐ Smoked
☐ Vaped
☐ Ingested
☐ Topical
☐ _____

CONTENT
____% CBD
____% THC
____% ____
____% ____
____% ____

VARIETY
☐ Indica
☐ Sativa
☐ Hybrid

Dose: _____ Smell / Taste: _____

Time to take effect: _____ Effect duration: _____

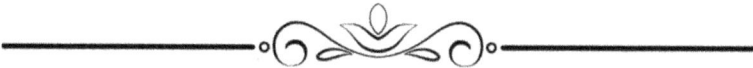

Reliefs

Pain:	① ② ③ ④ ⑤					Stress:	① ② ③ ④ ⑤			
Nausea:	① ② ③ ④ ⑤					Anxiety:	① ② ③ ④ ⑤			
Inflammation:	① ② ③ ④ ⑤					Insomnia:	① ② ③ ④ ⑤			
Appetite:	① ② ③ ④ ⑤					Depression:	① ② ③ ④ ⑤			

Other positive effects: _____

Adverse effects

Anxiety:	① ② ③ ④ ⑤					Dry Mouth:	① ② ③ ④ ⑤			
Munchies:	① ② ③ ④ ⑤					Fatigue:	① ② ③ ④ ⑤			

Other adverse effects: _____

Notes

My Rating: 🍁 🍁 🍁 🍁 🍁

DATE: ENTRY: 107

Strain:_____ Distributor:_____

PRICE: _____
TOTAL ACQUIRED: _____
PURCHASE DATE: _____
DISTRIBUTOR #: _____

description / notes

DOSAGE / INSTRUCTIONS	CERTIFICATE OF ANALYSIS	
	☐ Yes	☐ No

FORM	METHOD	CONTENT	VARIETY
☐ Flower	☐ Smoked	____% CBD	☐ Indica
☐ Edible	☐ Vaped	____% THC	☐ Sativa
☐ Oil	☐ Ingested	____% ____	☐ Hybrid
☐ Tincture	☐ Topical	____% ____	
☐ _____	☐ _____	____% ____	

Dose: _____   Smell / Taste: _____

Time to take effect: _____   Effect duration: _____

Reliefs

Pain: ① ② ③ ④ ⑤   Stress: ① ② ③ ④ ⑤
Nausea: ① ② ③ ④ ⑤   Anxiety: ① ② ③ ④ ⑤
Inflammation: ① ② ③ ④ ⑤   Insomnia: ① ② ③ ④ ⑤
Appetite: ① ② ③ ④ ⑤   Depression: ① ② ③ ④ ⑤

Other positive effects: _____

Adverse effects

Anxiety: ① ② ③ ④ ⑤   Dry Mouth: ① ② ③ ④ ⑤
Munchies: ① ② ③ ④ ⑤   Fatigue: ① ② ③ ④ ⑤

Other adverse effects: _____

Notes

My Rating:

Strain:_____ Distributor:_____

PRICE: _____
TOTAL ACQUIRED: _____
PURCHASE DATE: _____
DISTRIBUTOR #: _____

description / notes

DOSAGE / INSTRUCTIONS	CERTIFICATE OF ANALYSIS	
	☐ Yes	☐ No

FORM
☐ Flower
☐ Edible
☐ Oil
☐ Tincture
☐ _____

METHOD
☐ Smoked
☐ Vaped
☐ Ingested
☐ Topical
☐ _____

CONTENT
_____% CBD
_____% THC
_____% _____
_____% _____
_____% _____

VARIETY
☐ Indica
☐ Sativa
☐ Hybrid

Dose: _____ Smell / Taste: _____

Time to take effect: _____ Effect duration: _____

Reliefs
Pain: ① ② ③ ④ ⑤   Stress: ① ② ③ ④ ⑤
Nausea: ① ② ③ ④ ⑤   Anxiety: ① ② ③ ④ ⑤
Inflammation: ① ② ③ ④ ⑤   Insomnia: ① ② ③ ④ ⑤
Appetite: ① ② ③ ④ ⑤   Depression: ① ② ③ ④ ⑤

Other positive effects: _____

Adverse effects
Anxiety: ① ② ③ ④ ⑤   Dry Mouth: ① ② ③ ④ ⑤
Munchies: ① ② ③ ④ ⑤   Fatigue: ① ② ③ ④ ⑤

Other adverse effects: _____

Notes

My Rating: 🌿 🌿 🌿 🌿 🌿

Strain:_____ Distributor:_____

PRICE: _____
TOTAL ACQUIRED: _____
PURCHASE DATE: _____
DISTRIBUTOR #: _____

description / notes

DOSAGE / INSTRUCTIONS	CERTIFICATE OF ANALYSIS
	☐ Yes ☐ No

FORM
☐ Flower
☐ Edible
☐ Oil
☐ Tincture
☐ _____

METHOD
☐ Smoked
☐ Vaped
☐ Ingested
☐ Topical
☐ _____

CONTENT
_____% CBD
_____% THC
_____% _____
_____% _____
_____% _____

VARIETY
☐ Indica
☐ Sativa
☐ Hybrid

Dose: _____ Smell / Taste: _____

Time to take effect: _____ Effect duration: _____

Reliefs

Pain:	① ② ③ ④ ⑤	Stress:	① ② ③ ④ ⑤
Nausea:	① ② ③ ④ ⑤	Anxiety:	① ② ③ ④ ⑤
Inflammation:	① ② ③ ④ ⑤	Insomnia:	① ② ③ ④ ⑤
Appetite:	① ② ③ ④ ⑤	Depression:	① ② ③ ④ ⑤

Other positive effects: _____

Adverse effects

Anxiety:	① ② ③ ④ ⑤	Dry Mouth:	① ② ③ ④ ⑤
Munchies:	① ② ③ ④ ⑤	Fatigue:	① ② ③ ④ ⑤

Other adverse effects: _____

Notes

My Rating: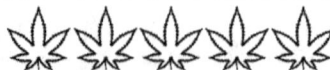

DATE:	ENTRY:	110

Strain:_____ Distributor:_____

PRICE: _____
TOTAL ACQUIRED: _____
PURCHASE DATE: _____
DISTRIBUTOR #: _____

description / notes

DOSAGE / INSTRUCTIONS	CERTIFICATE OF ANALYSIS	
	☐ Yes	☐ No

FORM
☐ Flower
☐ Edible
☐ Oil
☐ Tincture
☐ _____

METHOD
☐ Smoked
☐ Vaped
☐ Ingested
☐ Topical
☐ _____

CONTENT
_____% CBD
_____% THC
_____% _____
_____% _____
_____% _____

VARIETY
☐ Indica
☐ Sativa
☐ Hybrid

Dose: _____ Smell / Taste: _____

Time to take effect: _____ Effect duration: _____

Reliefs

Pain:	① ② ③ ④ ⑤	Stress:	① ② ③ ④ ⑤
Nausea:	① ② ③ ④ ⑤	Anxiety:	① ② ③ ④ ⑤
Inflammation:	① ② ③ ④ ⑤	Insomnia:	① ② ③ ④ ⑤
Appetite:	① ② ③ ④ ⑤	Depression:	① ② ③ ④ ⑤

Other positive effects: _____

Adverse effects

Anxiety:	① ② ③ ④ ⑤	Dry Mouth:	① ② ③ ④ ⑤
Munchies:	① ② ③ ④ ⑤	Fatigue:	① ② ③ ④ ⑤

Other adverse effects: _____

Notes

My Rating: 🍁 🍁 🍁 🍁 🍁

Strain:_____ Distributor:_____

PRICE: _____

TOTAL ACQUIRED: _____

PURCHASE DATE: _____

DISTRIBUTOR #: _____

description / notes

DOSAGE / INSTRUCTIONS	CERTIFICATE OF ANALYSIS	
	☐ Yes	☐ No

FORM
☐ Flower
☐ Edible
☐ Oil
☐ Tincture
☐ _____

METHOD
☐ Smoked
☐ Vaped
☐ Ingested
☐ Topical
☐ _____

CONTENT
_____% CBD
_____% THC
_____% _____
_____% _____
_____% _____

VARIETY
☐ Indica
☐ Sativa
☐ Hybrid

Dose: _____ Smell / Taste: _____

Time to take effect: _____ Effect duration: _____

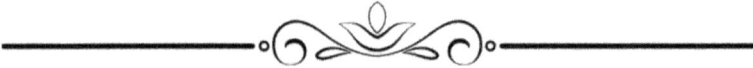

Reliefs

Pain:	① ② ③ ④ ⑤	Stress:	① ② ③ ④ ⑤
Nausea:	① ② ③ ④ ⑤	Anxiety:	① ② ③ ④ ⑤
Inflammation:	① ② ③ ④ ⑤	Insomnia:	① ② ③ ④ ⑤
Appetite:	① ② ③ ④ ⑤	Depression:	① ② ③ ④ ⑤

Other positive effects: _____

Adverse effects

Anxiety:	① ② ③ ④ ⑤	Dry Mouth:	① ② ③ ④ ⑤
Munchies:	① ② ③ ④ ⑤	Fatigue:	① ② ③ ④ ⑤

Other adverse effects: _____

Notes

My Rating: 🍁 🍁 🍁 🍁 🍁

Strain:_____ Distributor:_____

PRICE: _____
TOTAL ACQUIRED: _____
PURCHASE DATE: _____
DISTRIBUTOR #: _____

description / notes

DOSAGE / INSTRUCTIONS	CERTIFICATE OF ANALYSIS	
	☐ Yes	☐ No

FORM
☐ Flower
☐ Edible
☐ Oil
☐ Tincture
☐ _____

METHOD
☐ Smoked
☐ Vaped
☐ Ingested
☐ Topical
☐ _____

CONTENT
_____% CBD
_____% THC
_____% _____
_____% _____
_____% _____

VARIETY
☐ Indica
☐ Sativa
☐ Hybrid

Dose: _____ Smell / Taste: _____

Time to take effect: _____ Effect duration: _____

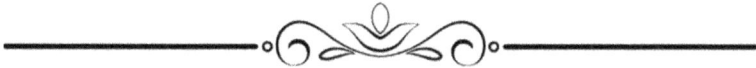

Reliefs

Pain:	① ② ③ ④ ⑤					Stress:	① ② ③ ④ ⑤		
Nausea:	① ② ③ ④ ⑤					Anxiety:	① ② ③ ④ ⑤		
Inflammation:	① ② ③ ④ ⑤					Insomnia:	① ② ③ ④ ⑤		
Appetite:	① ② ③ ④ ⑤					Depression:	① ② ③ ④ ⑤		

Other positive effects: _____

Adverse effects

Anxiety:	① ② ③ ④ ⑤	Dry Mouth:	① ② ③ ④ ⑤
Munchies:	① ② ③ ④ ⑤	Fatigue:	① ② ③ ④ ⑤

Other adverse effects: _____

Notes

My Rating: 🍁 🍁 🍁 🍁 🍁

DATE:	ENTRY:	113

Strain:_____ Distributor:_____

PRICE: _____

TOTAL ACQUIRED: _____

PURCHASE DATE: _____

DISTRIBUTOR #: _____

description / notes

DOSAGE / INSTRUCTIONS	CERTIFICATE OF ANALYSIS	
	☐ Yes	☐ No

FORM
☐ Flower

☐ Edible

☐ Oil

☐ Tincture

☐ _____

METHOD
☐ Smoked

☐ Vaped

☐ Ingested

☐ Topical

☐ _____

CONTENT
_____% CBD

_____% THC

_____% _____

_____% _____

_____% _____

VARIETY
☐ Indica

☐ Sativa

☐ Hybrid

Dose: _____ Smell / Taste: _____

Time to take effect: _____ Effect duration: _____

Reliefs

Pain:	① ② ③ ④ ⑤	Stress:	① ② ③ ④ ⑤
Nausea:	① ② ③ ④ ⑤	Anxiety:	① ② ③ ④ ⑤
Inflammation:	① ② ③ ④ ⑤	Insomnia:	① ② ③ ④ ⑤
Appetite:	① ② ③ ④ ⑤	Depression:	① ② ③ ④ ⑤

Other positive effects: _____

Adverse effects

Anxiety:	① ② ③ ④ ⑤	Dry Mouth:	① ② ③ ④ ⑤
Munchies:	① ② ③ ④ ⑤	Fatigue:	① ② ③ ④ ⑤

Other adverse effects: _____

Notes

My Rating:

Strain:_____ Distributor:_____

PRICE: _____
TOTAL ACQUIRED: _____
PURCHASE DATE: _____
DISTRIBUTOR #: _____

description / notes

DOSAGE / INSTRUCTIONS	CERTIFICATE OF ANALYSIS	
	☐ Yes	☐ No

FORM
☐ Flower
☐ Edible
☐ Oil
☐ Tincture
☐ _____

METHOD
☐ Smoked
☐ Vaped
☐ Ingested
☐ Topical
☐ _____

CONTENT
____% CBD
____% THC
____% ____
____% ____
____% ____

VARIETY
☐ Indica
☐ Sativa
☐ Hybrid

Dose: _____ Smell / Taste: _____

Time to take effect: _____ Effect duration: _____

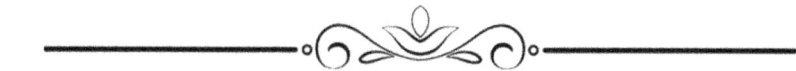

Reliefs

Pain:	① ② ③ ④ ⑤					Stress:	① ② ③ ④ ⑤			
Nausea:	① ② ③ ④ ⑤					Anxiety:	① ② ③ ④ ⑤			
Inflammation:	① ② ③ ④ ⑤					Insomnia:	① ② ③ ④ ⑤			
Appetite:	① ② ③ ④ ⑤					Depression:	① ② ③ ④ ⑤			

Other positive effects: _____

Adverse effects

Anxiety:	① ② ③ ④ ⑤					Dry Mouth:	① ② ③ ④ ⑤			
Munchies:	① ② ③ ④ ⑤					Fatigue:	① ② ③ ④ ⑤			

Other adverse effects: _____

Notes
_____

My Rating: 🌿 🌿 🌿 🌿 🌿

DATE:		ENTRY:	115

*Strain:*_____ *Distributor:*_____

PRICE: _____	*description / notes*
TOTAL ACQUIRED: _____	
PURCHASE DATE: _____	
DISTRIBUTOR #: _____	

DOSAGE / INSTRUCTIONS	CERTIFICATE OF ANALYSIS	
	☐ Yes	☐ No

FORM	METHOD	CONTENT	VARIETY
☐ Flower	☐ Smoked	_____% CBD	☐ Indica
☐ Edible	☐ Vaped	_____% THC	☐ Sativa
☐ Oil	☐ Ingested	_____% _____	☐ Hybrid
☐ Tincture	☐ Topical	_____% _____	
☐ _____	☐ _____	_____% _____	

Dose: _____ Smell / Taste: _____

Time to take effect: _____ Effect duration: _____

Reliefs

Pain:	①	②	③	④	⑤	Stress:	①	②	③	④	⑤
Nausea:	①	②	③	④	⑤	Anxiety:	①	②	③	④	⑤
Inflammation:	①	②	③	④	⑤	Insomnia:	①	②	③	④	⑤
Appetite:	①	②	③	④	⑤	Depression:	①	②	③	④	⑤

Other positive effects: _____

Adverse effects

Anxiety:	①	②	③	④	⑤	Dry Mouth:	①	②	③	④	⑤
Munchies:	①	②	③	④	⑤	Fatigue:	①	②	③	④	⑤

Other adverse effects: _____

Notes

My Rating: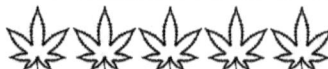

Strain:_____ Distributor:_____

PRICE: _____
TOTAL ACQUIRED: _____
PURCHASE DATE: _____
DISTRIBUTOR #: _____

description / notes

DOSAGE / INSTRUCTIONS	CERTIFICATE OF ANALYSIS	
	☐ Yes	☐ No

FORM
☐ Flower
☐ Edible
☐ Oil
☐ Tincture
☐ _____

METHOD
☐ Smoked
☐ Vaped
☐ Ingested
☐ Topical
☐ _____

CONTENT
____% CBD
____% THC
____% ____
____% ____
____% ____

VARIETY
☐ Indica
☐ Sativa
☐ Hybrid

Dose: _____   Smell / Taste: _____

Time to take effect: _____   Effect duration: _____

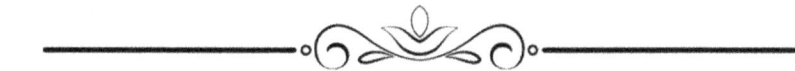

Reliefs

Pain:	① ② ③ ④ ⑤	Stress:	① ② ③ ④ ⑤
Nausea:	① ② ③ ④ ⑤	Anxiety:	① ② ③ ④ ⑤
Inflammation:	① ② ③ ④ ⑤	Insomnia:	① ② ③ ④ ⑤
Appetite:	① ② ③ ④ ⑤	Depression:	① ② ③ ④ ⑤

Other positive effects: _____

Adverse effects

Anxiety:	① ② ③ ④ ⑤	Dry Mouth:	① ② ③ ④ ⑤
Munchies:	① ② ③ ④ ⑤	Fatigue:	① ② ③ ④ ⑤

Other adverse effects: _____

Notes

_____

My Rating: 🍁 🍁 🍁 🍁 🍁

Strain:_____ Distributor:_____

PRICE: _____

TOTAL ACQUIRED: _____

PURCHASE DATE: _____

DISTRIBUTOR #: _____

description / notes

DOSAGE / INSTRUCTIONS	CERTIFICATE OF ANALYSIS	
	☐ Yes	☐ No

FORM
☐ Flower
☐ Edible
☐ Oil
☐ Tincture
☐ _____

METHOD
☐ Smoked
☐ Vaped
☐ Ingested
☐ Topical
☐ _____

CONTENT
_____% CBD
_____% THC
_____% _____
_____% _____
_____% _____

VARIETY
☐ Indica
☐ Sativa
☐ Hybrid

Dose: _____ Smell / Taste: _____

Time to take effect: _____ Effect duration: _____

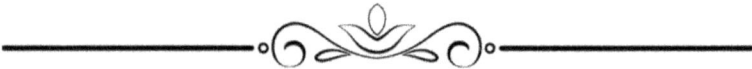

Reliefs

Pain:	①	②	③	④	⑤	Stress:	①	②	③	④	⑤
Nausea:	①	②	③	④	⑤	Anxiety:	①	②	③	④	⑤
Inflammation:	①	②	③	④	⑤	Insomnia:	①	②	③	④	⑤
Appetite:	①	②	③	④	⑤	Depression:	①	②	③	④	⑤

Other positive effects: _____

Adverse effects

Anxiety:	①	②	③	④	⑤	Dry Mouth:	①	②	③	④	⑤
Munchies:	①	②	③	④	⑤	Fatigue:	①	②	③	④	⑤

Other adverse effects: _____

Notes

My Rating:

DATE:	ENTRY:	118

Strain:_____ Distributor:_____

PRICE: _____

TOTAL ACQUIRED: _____

PURCHASE DATE: _____

DISTRIBUTOR #: _____

description / notes

DOSAGE / INSTRUCTIONS	CERTIFICATE OF ANALYSIS	
	☐ Yes	☐ No

FORM
☐ Flower
☐ Edible
☐ Oil
☐ Tincture
☐ _____

METHOD
☐ Smoked
☐ Vaped
☐ Ingested
☐ Topical
☐ _____

CONTENT
_____% CBD
_____% THC
_____% _____
_____% _____
_____% _____

VARIETY
☐ Indica
☐ Sativa
☐ Hybrid

Dose: _____ Smell / Taste: _____

Time to take effect: _____ Effect duration: _____

Reliefs

Pain: ① ② ③ ④ ⑤   Stress: ① ② ③ ④ ⑤

Nausea: ① ② ③ ④ ⑤   Anxiety: ① ② ③ ④ ⑤

Inflammation: ① ② ③ ④ ⑤   Insomnia: ① ② ③ ④ ⑤

Appetite: ① ② ③ ④ ⑤   Depression: ① ② ③ ④ ⑤

Other positive effects: _____

Adverse effects

Anxiety: ① ② ③ ④ ⑤   Dry Mouth: ① ② ③ ④ ⑤

Munchies: ① ② ③ ④ ⑤   Fatigue: ① ② ③ ④ ⑤

Other adverse effects: _____

Notes

My Rating:

DATE:		ENTRY:	119

Strain:_____ Distributor:_____

PRICE: _____

TOTAL ACQUIRED: _____

PURCHASE DATE: _____

DISTRIBUTOR #: _____

description / notes

DOSAGE / INSTRUCTIONS	CERTIFICATE OF ANALYSIS	
	☐ Yes	☐ No

FORM	METHOD	CONTENT	VARIETY
☐ Flower	☐ Smoked	_____% CBD	☐ Indica
☐ Edible	☐ Vaped	_____% THC	☐ Sativa
☐ Oil	☐ Ingested	_____% _____	☐ Hybrid
☐ Tincture	☐ Topical	_____% _____	
☐ _____	☐ _____	_____% _____	

Dose: _____ Smell / Taste: _____

Time to take effect: _____ Effect duration: _____

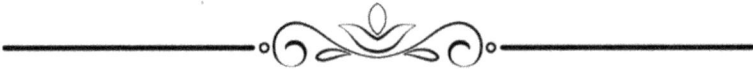

Reliefs

Pain:	①②③④⑤	Stress:	①②③④⑤
Nausea:	①②③④⑤	Anxiety:	①②③④⑤
Inflammation:	①②③④⑤	Insomnia:	①②③④⑤
Appetite:	①②③④⑤	Depression:	①②③④⑤

Other positive effects: _____

Adverse effects

Anxiety:	①②③④⑤	Dry Mouth:	①②③④⑤
Munchies:	①②③④⑤	Fatigue:	①②③④⑤

Other adverse effects: _____

Notes

My Rating: 🍁🍁🍁🍁🍁

Strain:_____ Distributor:_____

PRICE: _____
TOTAL ACQUIRED: _____
PURCHASE DATE: _____
DISTRIBUTOR #: _____

description / notes

DOSAGE / INSTRUCTIONS	CERTIFICATE OF ANALYSIS	
	☐ Yes	☐ No

FORM
☐ Flower
☐ Edible
☐ Oil
☐ Tincture
☐ _____

METHOD
☐ Smoked
☐ Vaped
☐ Ingested
☐ Topical
☐ _____

CONTENT
_____% CBD
_____% THC
_____% _____
_____% _____
_____% _____

VARIETY
☐ Indica
☐ Sativa
☐ Hybrid

Dose: _____ Smell / Taste: _____

Time to take effect: _____ Effect duration: _____

Reliefs

Pain:	①	②	③	④	⑤	Stress:	①	②	③	④	⑤
Nausea:	①	②	③	④	⑤	Anxiety:	①	②	③	④	⑤
Inflammation:	①	②	③	④	⑤	Insomnia:	①	②	③	④	⑤
Appetite:	①	②	③	④	⑤	Depression:	①	②	③	④	⑤

Other positive effects: _____

Adverse effects

Anxiety:	①	②	③	④	⑤	Dry Mouth:	①	②	③	④	⑤
Munchies:	①	②	③	④	⑤	Fatigue:	①	②	③	④	⑤

Other adverse effects: _____

Notes

My Rating: 🍁 🍁 🍁 🍁 🍁

Notes

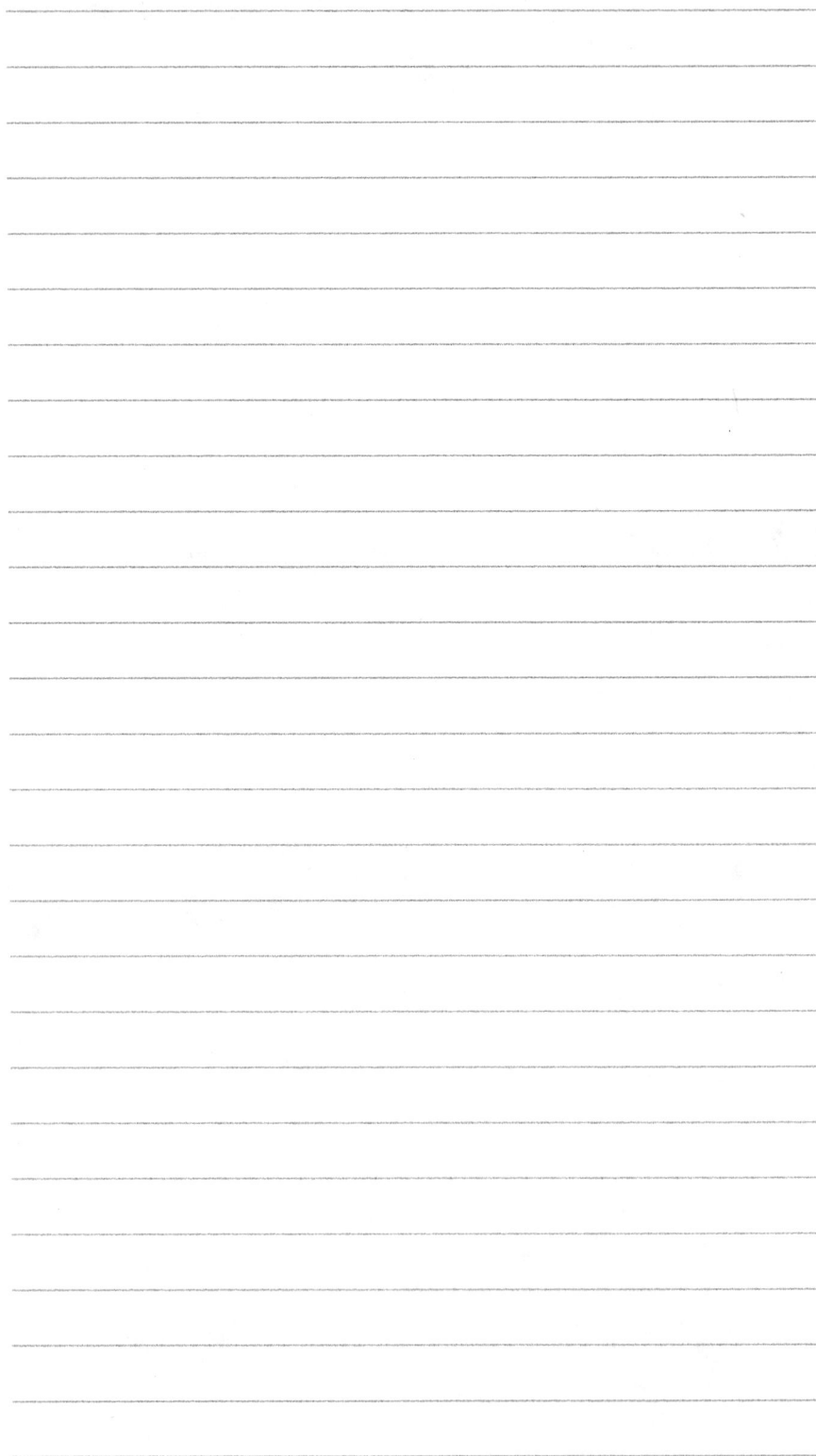